Marna's Corner

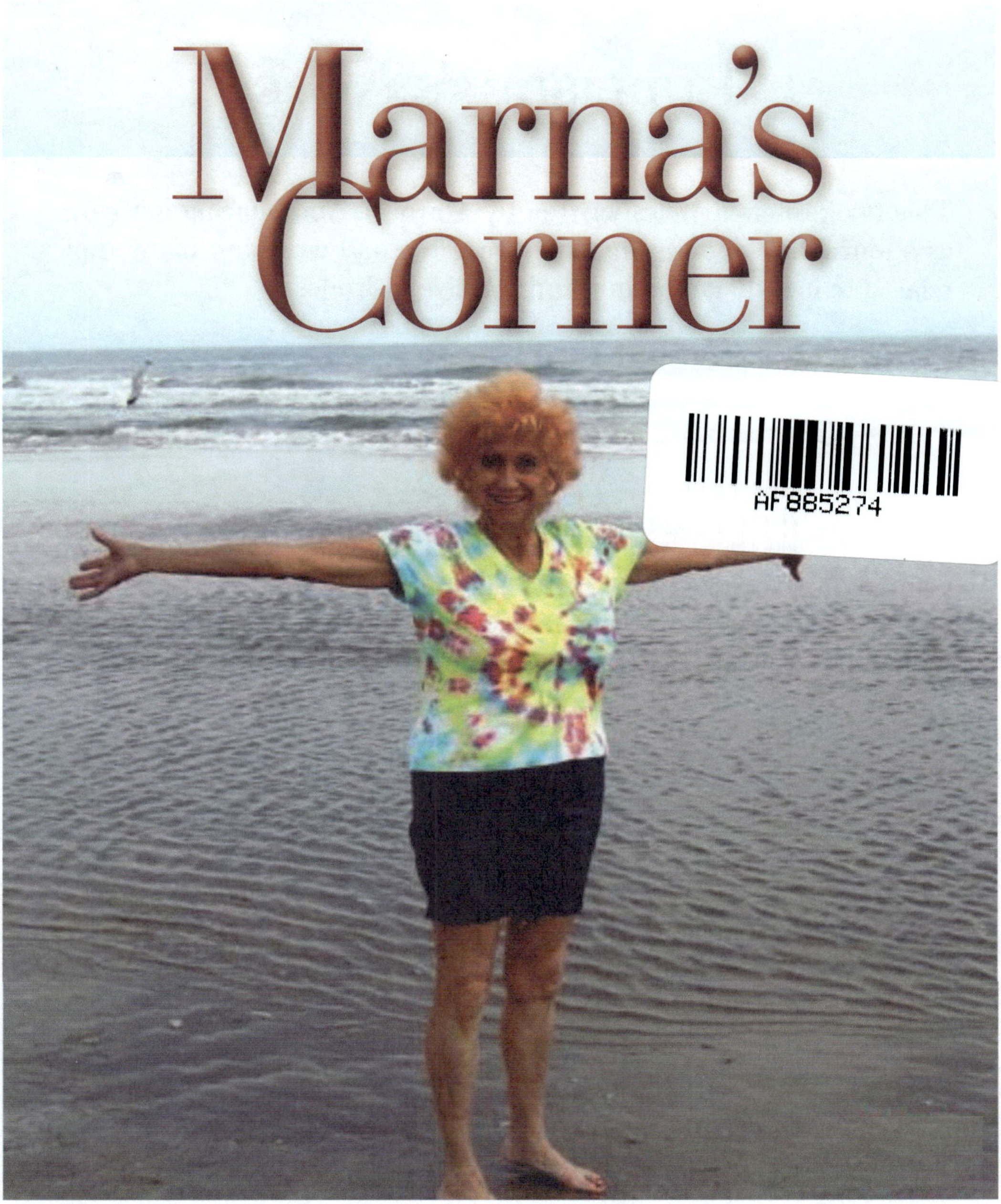

Marna L'Amie

TREATY OAK PUBLISHERS

Publisher's Note

This book offers articles written by Marna L'Amie during her career as a journalist. She was an avid researcher and writer on many topics related to health, gardening, and positive attitudes.

Printed and published in the United States of America

TREATY OAK PUBLISHERS

ISBN-978-1-959127-32-1

Dedication

to my uncle, Jerry Robins,
who fervently believed in Mom and her writings

to the memory of her beloved late husband, Bill L'Amie

and to the blessed memory of Marna Robins L'Amie

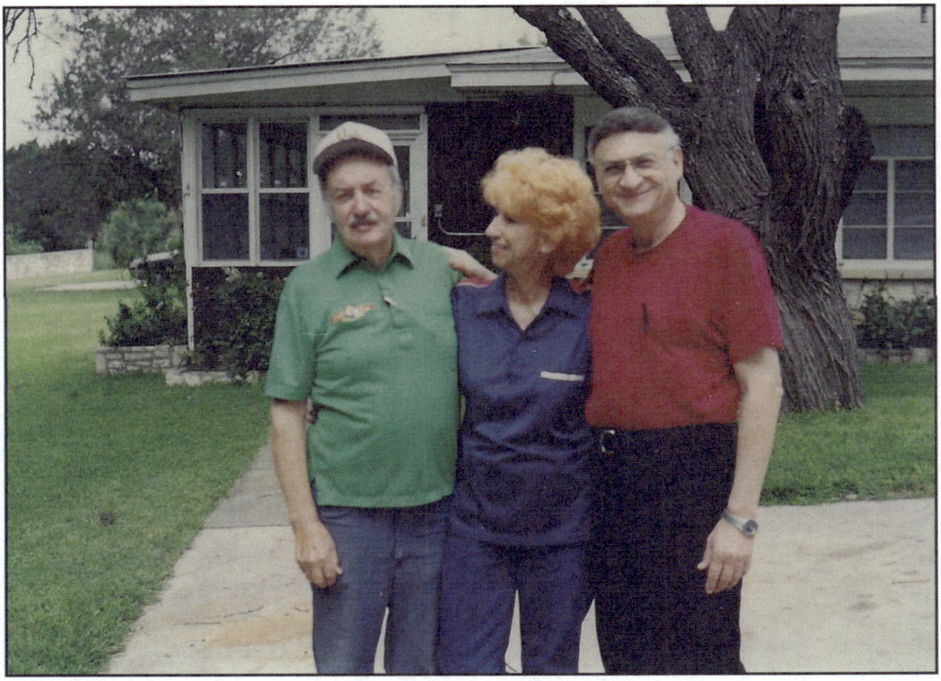

Table of Contents

Introduction

My mother, Marna Robins (Franklin) L'Amie, was an incredible woman—a larger than life, passionate, brilliant, extremely outspoken, loving human being. Originally a raven-haired beauty, she became a "reddish/orange-head" while attempting to bleach her graying hair blonde. Mom was a prolific writer, lecturer, teacher, and voracious reader and researcher.

Besides being a dedicated wife and mother of four children, she loved nothing more than passing along her knowledge to those who might benefit from it. My childhood home was always filled with my sister's friends—whom she tutored in algebra—Jewish adult study groups (with our father, Jack Franklin), or simply our teenaged friends, who knew Mom would honestly answer questions and/or discuss delicate subjects.

Mom attended the University of Oklahoma for about two years, studying art and fashion design, and later, as an adult, attended McMurry College in Abilene, Texas. She never obtained a degree but continued to be a lifetime learner. In the early 1970's, when women were rarely involved in math or the sciences, she took courses and worked in computer programming, as well as educating herself about auto mechanics and becoming a successful car salesperson. She taught courses at a business school, held seminars (along with her second husband, Bill L'Amie) on positive thinking and self-esteem, wrote about health and gardening, and spoke to churches and college classes about Judaism.

Marna wrote advertising copy for radio, magazine, and newspaper ads. Incredibly intelligent, highly competitive at Scrabble, Mom answered crossword puzzles in pen (challenging my husband as to the necessity of using a pencil), was a Master gardener, a fabulous hostess, excellent cook, and a talented seamstress.

Although she was concerned about nutrition and health her entire life, in later life she became an evangelist for natural remedies for health issues instead of pharmaceutical solutions. She wrote a monthly column for *Living Naturally First*, a magazine concerned with health and gardening.

Those articles were written between 2010-2016.

This book is a compilation of most of her articles. Also included are some of her inspired writings for a weekly column entitled "Marna's Corner," published in the Gladewater Mirror.

My siblings and I joke about Mom's intense passion about health and food, sometimes embarrassing us by cornering friends and family to lecture them on the evils of taking statins or the healing benefits of coconut oil. Truth be told, though, she would be pleased to learn that in recent years, positive research has substantiated many of her strong beliefs.

More than anything else, my mother wanted to do "tikkun olam," a Hebrew phrase meaning "to help the world." Although she left this earthly world in April 2016, we hope her influence will live on through these writings.

Many doctors and researchers were quoted in this book. Marna was not a physician, but a well-read and industrious researcher. Her advice should only be taken as such.

Melanie Cox

Marna's Corner

Program your mind with positive thoughts, and you direct it into bringing you what you want.

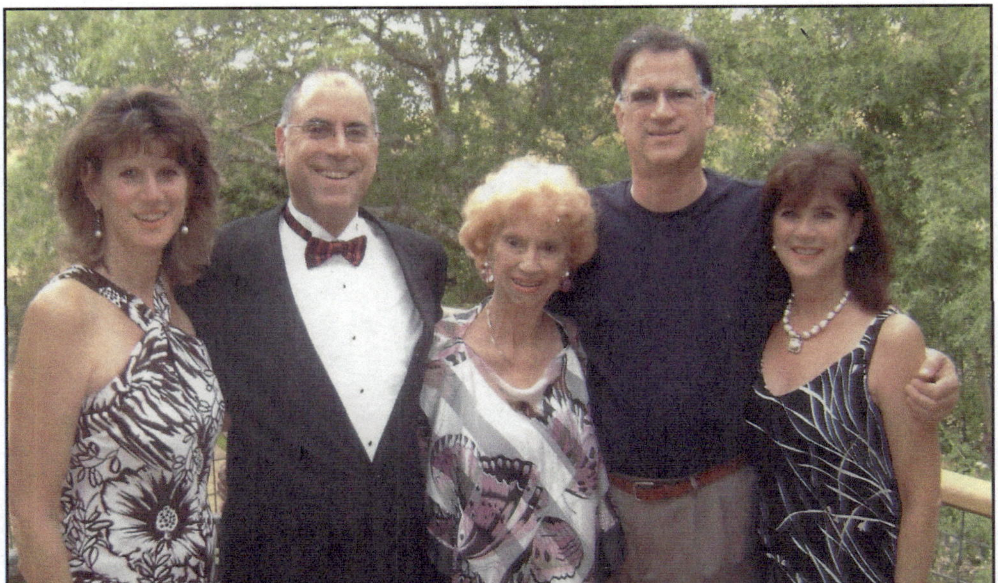

Marna and her children
Melanie Cox, Bram Franklin, Marna, Richard Franklin, and Lynda Furgatch

Motivation and Positive Thinking

This column is always concerned with nutrition, ways to prevent disease and illness, build a strong immune system, and it also covers other various methods of natural healing. There are many aspects of wellness; happiness and joy are two of them. Relieving stress and peace of mind is another. I taught "Motivation" and "Positive Thinking" and wrote articles on the subject in newspapers and magazines in East Texas for twenty-five years before moving to the Austin area. I have decided to use this space this month for several columns that are over thirty years old... but just as powerful as they were when first published. Following are some excerpts from those columns.

"A few months ago, we had the most ferocious, the loudest, the worst lightning and thunder storm I have ever seen or heard in my entire life.

And the next morning was calm, beautiful, with blue skies and little white puffs of clouds floating here and there.

What a demonstration that God promises peace, calm, and beauty. If we just wait a little while, knowing the most terrible of storms is only a prelude, a passing noise... and nothing to cause fear.

Just listen and watch and wait for morning.

❦ ❦ ❦

Miracles are called coincidences by the uninitiated. After all, what do we consider a 'miracle'?

- an impossibility.
- a happening that we cannot affect.
- a very propitious event that we did not expect.
- a 'what if' or 'if only' occurrence.

We hear of miracles occasionally in the lives of others (and really disbelieve them in our inner mind); but we cannot conceive of them close to home in our own lives.

But… they… do… happen… every day! We just have to be aware… and, we must stop refuting and negating miracles because we do not believe.

Miracles happen every day, we just have to look for them.

There is no hurry, push, or force on the prosperous plane of life. Take one step at a time each day, and do it calmly with no haste, worry, or fear. The moment you begin to hurry, you become fearful… the prelude to failure. When you realize that you are forcing a result, stop! Fix your mind's eye on what you hope to achieve, and then give thanks that you are receiving it.

Fear is the greatest barrier in our lives! During World War II, President Franklin Delano Roosevelt said, "The only thing we have to fear is fear itself."

And he was right. When fear gets a hold on us, our stomach knots up, our hands get clammy, some of us get dizzy, and we cannot function. If it comes in the middle of the night, it is a thousand times worse. And fear, like any other emotion, can be overcome. Children are virtually fearless. Parents instill fear in us, some necessary…" don't put your hand on that hot stove burner" …and some virtually damaging… "that doggy is going to bite you!" We feel and adopt our parents' subconscious fears, too. We learn so much by the time we are five or six years old, learning that takes us a lifetime to overcome. We are very impressionable in our early years and carry those feelings around for life unless we reprogram ourselves. *It can be done*!

You must just decide, as I did, that life is not worth living with so much fear. It takes the joy out of everything. It is said that 95% of all we fear *never* happens! I found that to be true. I realized that most of the time I went through all of that excruciating fear and worry ahead of time, and then nothing happened, and all of it was needless. If the feared event did occur, I felt bad enough at the time, without all the previous days or weeks of immobilizing fear. Fear doesn't change a thing; it just brings pain. I just decided I would hope for the best, not fear for the worst, and I got on with my life.

If I could, so can you.

❦ ❦ ❦

When you walk into a dark room, there is no need to push all of the darkness out; all you must do is turn a light on.

Every one of us is seeking LOVE and APPROVAL with a capital L and a capital A! If we feel loved, if we feel that those around us completely approve of what we do and who we are, we are happy, well-adjusted, whole human beings. If, on the other hand, we lack someone to love us; if we think we do not have the approval of others... that they do not think will of us; we are absolutely miserable, depressed, even physically ill at times. Love *really* does make the world go round!

Money and material possessions are wonderful to have. We can do many fun and happy things with no monetary worries. But without anyone to love us or approve of us, it is a v.e.r.y l.o.n.e.l.y existence.

We were created in Love, and we are meant to give it to others and to receive it in kind.

❦ ❦ ❦

All life, all matter is made up of energy. You are a *forcefield* of energy. You can direct that energy anywhere, in any manner you choose. The secret is in knowing how to direct it! You are directing it every moment, consciously or unconsciously, to your benefit or to your detriment. Program your mind with positive thoughts, and you direct it into bringing you that which you want. If you do not *cancel out* negative thoughts that steal into your head, or if you unconsciously let anything and everything that enters, stay... you are letting go of control and allowing that which you do *not* want into your life.

The only thing you can control in this life are your thoughts. The mind can only dwell on one thing at a time. Control what you think. Be a guardian at the door. Bring only good into your life. Health, Success, Love, Joy, and Peace of Mind are yours with mental discipline.

❦ ❦ ❦

My husband, William L'Amie, who lectured on Positive Thinking at my side, wrote this column.

"The leaders, the winners, the DO IT NOW PEOPLE... whatever

banner these people run with in the RACE THROUGH LIFE… they have one thing in common. THEY ARE EXCEPTIONAL LISTENERS!

They ask and ask and ask questions. They are not so interested in telling you what they know as they are in finding out what you know. Leaders have developed emotional filters for personal growth and success. They have an OPEN MIND. People with an OPEN MIND are willing to explore THEIR OWN BELIEFS!

Good listening will help us make better decisions. Asking meaningful questions can open a new world. Are YOU A GOOD LISTENER?"

Appreciation

We take our daily happenings for granted, never thinking what else could have transpired. We wake up in the morning, eat our breakfast, clear up the house and kitchen, and do whatever errands we had for today, taking for granted we can get in our car to transport us to wherever we have to go, and to whatever we have to do.

What if we cannot get out of bed because we are ill, or have had surgery, and have been told that we will get better with time… just have patience, and we will get back into our usual form? Do you know it takes three weeks for the trauma of surgery to clear out of the body? Do you know it takes one month's time for every hour under anesthesia to completely regenerate? Who knew how long it would take for the anesthesia to leave our bodies?

Do you know that while you are in the hospital, four, five, six days or more, you cannot get out of bed without calling a nurse first; that an alarm will ring if you are able to get up? We take for granted that we will continue to move, act, and think in the normal, healthy manner we have been used to for so many years.

When you return home, it will take at least four weeks, (or more), to be able to drive a car. What has been your freedom to come and go as you wish, to continue life as it has been, to see people or businesses to complete your day is no longer a reality. Without the ability to drive, your car sits in your driveway, and you sit in your home. You are a prisoner without the ability to go anywhere!

Think about the freedom you have with the ability to think clearly (no brain fog), and to move about as, when, and where you please. We take this all for granted… until it is no longer a viable ability.

If you live alone, you need someone to take care of your meals, your laundry, your kitchen, your mail, your groceries, etc. And you are mostly confined to bed because of weakness. You are lucky if you belong to libraries where you can borrow books to read, because otherwise you are bored to death, having no interest in anything but getting well and being free to live your usual full life. Unless friends or family come by each day, no one is there to communicate with you or to help you fill your needs. It is a very lonely existence!

Then is when you figure out that you were not appreciative of daily abilities… that if you wish to go to the bathroom, you just get up and walk into the room you wish… no thought of "may I"? We do not appreciate the 'little' things we are used to, minute by minute, until we no longer have the ability to pursue the 'little' things. Then they become 'b.i.g' things.

When we need help, friends do show up, happy to help with our needs. Do you appreciate your friends? Do you help them, usually without considering whether they will help you when you are in need? Again, let them know how much you enjoy them, as a daily thought, not just when you are in need. They will enjoy hearing you say so. We rarely tell others how happy we are to know them… it just isn't usually done. But think how happy you would be to hear that from friends.

Wake up this morning. Keep an eye on everything you do when you rise. Think how tied down you would be if you could not get out of bed. Every action you take this morning, realize how shorted you would be if you could not take that action. That is when you will understand and appreciate your ability to move, think, and attend to normal, everyday situations, instead of being hamstrung.

Give 'Thanks' you are well and will stay well. Do not take it for granted.

Gardening and Soil

PLANT LIFE:

In the last century, we have burned up more than 90% of the organic matter in many of our soils through tilling, applying chemicals, and clearing plant residue without allowing organic matter to decompose. Conventional gardening has largely ignored organic matter and the resulting plant life has lost nutrients.

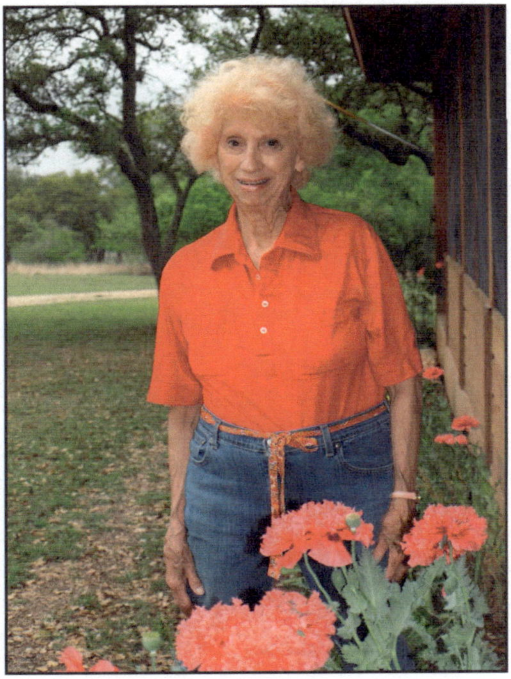

Healthy Soil Equals Nutritious Food

Nutritious food has natural health properties that pharmaceutical companies isolate and compound, causing the harmful side effects of their drugs. Instead of using all the synergistic varied parts of a healthy, natural plant, only specific parts are separated and incorporated into their patents.

Nature has made the whole food and its component parts work together to build our immunity to disease and illness... that is called HEALTH! That is the source of our energy, our vitality, our sexuality, our happiness, and our joy. We should be happy beings, not fearful, anxious, sleepless, worried, tired humans. We should awaken in the morning eager to go, finishing all of the tasks we had planned to complete. Food that has been raised in nutrient dense (rich) soil that has not been depleted with chemical salt fertilizers (synthetic, man-made) and pesticides, herbicides and insecticides is the prime factor in our health.

In the book, *Building Soil Naturally*, by Phil Nauta, he explains that vigorous, more pest-resistant vegetables, flowers, and ornamental plants need complete and balanced nutrients... far beyond the simplistic, unbalanced concept of NPK (nitrogen, phosphorus, potash). The microbes, bacteria, fungi, protozoa, nematodes, yeasts, algae, carbon humates, insects, and animals in and around the garden actually create the plant's ability to flourish. His six steps to creating healthy soil, and thus, healthy plants are these:

1. Water

PLANT LIFE: Our plants are made of water, and they need it for photosynthesis and cooling. Insects, earthworms, and microbes all need water. What is often overlooked is that all living species in our garden need water. If city water is used, chlorine, fluoride, and other toxins are used to clean it up before it gets to our system. That is why capturing rainwater is so important. To protect our water, we can start by not using pesticides, chemical fertilizers, and genetically modified products (GMO'S).

HUMAN LIFE: Water is essential to life. Not only do we drink it, but also we are made of it. You will see how our lives parallel plant life in what we consume, and whether we are aware of and avoid the toxins that are present.

2. Organic Matter

PLANT LIFE: In the last century, we have burned up more than 90% of the organic matter in many of our soils through tilling, applying chemicals, and clearing plant residue without allowing organic matter to decompose. Humus is the ultimate goal, but a supply of fresh organic residue as food and shelter for microbes and animals is also necessary as this residue is broken down, carbon dioxide becomes available for plants. Conventional gardening has largely ignored organic matter and the resulting plant life has lost nutrients.

HUMAN LIFE: Our immune systems have suffered in the same way over the past 75-80 years, from the processed food we ingest that has much less nutrient content and contains preservatives, coloring, synthetics, sugars, salt, and many additives of which we are not even aware. Only 25% of our populace are healthy. Others have various ailments that did not happen yesterday or last week, but over a number of years of poor lifestyles. Our salvation would be in eating REAL FOOD, buying organic food, cooking our own meals, exercising our bodies, getting a full night's sleep, and a cessation of smoking and/or heavy drinking.

3. Microbial Inoculants

Microbes make our soil healthy, feed and protect our plants, and clean our water. They help control weeds, insects, and diseases. There are a number of ways to inoculate our soil and garden with microbes.

Mycorrhizal fungi greatly improve soil characteristics and are among the most important microbes that form relationships with plants. Compost mimics nature and speeds it up by quickly increasing the number and diversity of microbes and macro-fauna (earthworms, grubs, etc.), organic matter content, and nutrients in our soil. Aerated compost tea extracts and multiplies an astonishing number and diversity of beneficial, active, aerobic microbes and can inoculate the leaves of plants, too.

4. Supplementing Nutrients

PLANT LIFE: The next step is fertilization. Microbes and plants need nutrients. We want fertilizers derived from naturally mined rock and from plants… and we want to make sure they are not from genetically modified crops. A mix of both dry and liquid fertilizers achieve short and long-term goals. And they must be applied throughout the growing season.

HUMAN LIFE: Since our food nutrients have been slowly depleted with conventional agriculture soil practices over the past 75-80 years, we definitely need supplemental nutrients to complement our diets. We need to add the missing vitamins and minerals and trace nutrients. Seventy-five percent of our populace are deficient in Vitamin C and Vitamin D3. The harmful trans fats—corn, soybean, canola, safflower, sunflower, and cottonseed— make it a necessity to take Omega-3 oils. Sea vegetation brims over with dense nutrients that our depleted soils lack.

Each one of us must research what our individual bodies require.

5. Bio stimulants and Micronutrients

PLANT LIFE: There are more than eighty elements, many of which are important in small amounts as catalysts and enzymes in the soil and plants. Examples are iron, manganese, copper, molybdenum, and selenium. Our food supply is severely lacking in most of these, and our health is suffering as a result.

HUMAN LIFE: Our bodies need enzymes and amino acids, as well as vitamins and minerals. And again, our food supply is lacking in these, and our health is suffering as a result.

6. Energy

PLANT LIFE: Energy comes from microbes and animals, water, air, plant roots, nutrients, and from the interactions of all of these things.

HUMAN LIFE: Our energy also comes from all the various sources of organic foods and all of the nutrients therein.

Real Manure… or Synthetic

This will be a very hard column for most of you to read. Since I am unleashing and exposing bold TRUTH, not general marketing blitz, I will shock most of you.

How many of you think about the steak you just ate… or the chicken cutlets…or goat ribs… or lamb chops: where and how they were raised, what they ate… if the soil that produced their food and sustenance was enriched by REAL MANURE (real cow, chicken, goat, or lamb "feces"), not petroleum-based synthetic manure that offered absolutely no nutrients, just empty calories???

I could cry… I do cry when my seminar students, from twenty years to seventy-five years, want to know how to fix their arthritis, diabetes, headaches and migraines, indigestive diseases such as colitis, acid reflux and bloating, asthma and allergies, heart problems, lost memory, cancer, imbalance, lack of energy and strength… and many more physical or mental problems… but are completely unaware that the cause is what they've been eating for years! I have been saying for the past five years I have been writing for *Living Naturally First*: YOU ARE WHAT YOU EAT!"

The processed food we buy in our grocery stores has been altered since 1950 to lower their cost and make billions of $$$ for the producers. Actual nutrient value has been lost from lack of animal manure that has been exchanged for synthetic petroleum fertilizer, causing the loss each year of thousands of acres of producing soil per state. (After World War II, the petroleum that produced bombs and bullets was no longer needed: instead, it was switched to producing this synthetic fertilizer and harming our soil.)

How many of you ask if the animal whose meat you purchase has been grass-fed most of its life? The majority of our cattle spend the last eight months of life in an enclosed feed-lot, standing with insecticides and pesticides at their feet (in order to counteract the insects and mess there), are fed genetically-modified corn (cows do not eat corn, they eat grass and hay), and are shot up with antibiotics and growth hormones. Do you realize that animal's meat has been altered? Doesn't that meat sound appetizing?

How many of you ask, as I do, "What did you spray your vegetables… or fruit with?" Have you decided Organic produce costs too much, and you can wash off the pesticides, insecticides, and herbicides? It cannot all be washed off. It penetrates the skin deeper into the flesh.

Do you realize how expensive it is to fight the diseases contracted from these harmful foods? How many dollars do you pay your doctor, over and above hospitalization charges, to give you pharmaceutical drugs or perform surgery needed for hope of healing? And are you aware that the drugs you use just put off the immediate problem and cause a need for more drugs? Most of the old folks who end up in nursing homes are over-prescribed with an immense variety of drugs, some of which do not react well with others.

Are you just too busy and tired after a day's work to select healthy food? Because that is the cure for your ailments, not drugs. Or, since both adults in a home now work, is it easier to pick up whatever the butcher shop or produce department has, or buy food already cooked and processed (with the additives, preservatives, coloring, synthetic, and addictive products within) than to bother with intelligent and healthy choices?

If you don't want to change your habits and your lifestyle, then you pay with illness.

I tell my students, "It is your choice."

Soil, Plant, and Animal Fertility Our Health Cycle

Why is organic food healthier than conventional food?

Great masses of our population are in the dark about what "organic" means. The simple truth is that plants grown in fertile soil provide nutritious content to the one who consumes it. When an animal eats those nutritious plants, their meat is also nutritious. When we eat the animal that eats this plant life, we also gain nutrition.

Nutrition is energy. Energy is health. When we lack energy, we are ill. Our immune system falters, we are ripe for disease, we feel lethargic.

Most Americans are not aware that since World War II, the chemicals we used for explosives were redirected to synthetic chemical fertilizers, pesticides, herbicides, and insecticides. Where, before the 1940's, we used traditional manures, minerals, composts, mulches, and natural supplements such as bonemeal, bloodmeal, molasses, limestone, and ashes to enrich the soil, now the artificial, synthetic, chemical products have taken precedence. The chemical corporations paid for the expensive advertising and marketing systems that convinced farmers and gardeners to believe their processes were the new and better way to go. For sixty years, we have been pouring inorganic, chemical agricultural products into our soil. It has taken a toll in turning thousands of acres of healthy soil into desert lands, not only here in America, but over the entire world. California loses 10,000 acres a year. Worldwide, we lose 26,000 acres daily.

Malcolm Beck, the southwest's foremost composter, farmer, and gardener, says in his book, *Lessons in Nature*, "In order for a plant to be properly fed, whether with chemical or natural fertilizer, the microbial life in the soil must first process the fertilizer into a substance and release it in the correct amounts that are perfect for a plant to absorb. In order for the microbes to perform this service, they must have energy. They are not in the presence of sunlight, nor do they have chlorophyll like higher plants, so the microbes must get their energy from decaying plant or animal matter in the soil.

A bag of organic fertilizer has all the carbon/energy to meet the needs of the soil microbes. A bag of chemical fertilizer has no energy. If organic matter is not already present in the soil, the chemicals can quickly become stressful, even toxic, to the plants. This makes plants susceptible to disease and insect problems.

Chemical fertilizers can do nothing more than grow a plant. They do not build or sustain healthy soil. Organic fertilizers contain the energy and many other things that continually build soil fertility, crumb structure, increased water holding capacity, food for all beneficial soil life, condition the soil, and contribute to the hundreds of other yet-unknown things that cause a plant to grow healthy and perfect.

"Only healthy and perfectly grown plants can feed and support healthy animal and human life."

Thus, it is as simple as ABC!!!

The microbes in the soil must be fed to be active. Carbon-rich organic waste, which is composed of once living plant and animal life returned to the soil, provides the energy the microbes need to process the fertilizer. Missing from chemical fertilizers is the energy the soil life needs to process the fertilizer. Without this energy, an endless cycle of soil exhaustion is begun and energy is depleted. Again, we gain more acres of desert and have less stored water.

The plants that are raised in fertile soil give us the vitamins, minerals, enzymes, and amino acids needed for our health. Eating spinach or oranges from depleted soil gives us empty calories, not healthy, fulfilled bodies.

The animals that are pasture-fed and eat nutritious plant-life are also healthy and give us nutrition when we consume their meat. The animals raised in feedlots on corn and soy (a great percentage of which are genetically modified) that cows do not naturally eat and are fed bovine growth hormones and antibiotics and are sprayed with pesticides, are not healthy specimens, so we get no nutrition from them. Their meat decreases our immune system. (The fat from feedlot animals is Omega-6, which has been added to so many of our processed foods for at least forty years, is so out of proportion to Omega-3, it harms our organs by oxidizing them.)

To sum up:

- Soil is made fertile and nutritious from organic fertilizers.
- Plants are nutritious if grown in fertile soil.
- Animals get healthy and nutritious from eating fertile plants.
- We get our health and nutrition from eating these plants and animals.

Your life and your health and longevity *depend* upon your understanding these truths. Your life is truly in your choices. I cannot stress that enough! Don't only read what I have written, HEAR IT, realize the content of what you are reading, USE the knowledge.

Health is energy, vitality, happiness, sexuality, joyfulness, balance, and a lack of aches, pains, and weakness.

My sources for this column are *Lessons in Nature*, by Malcom Beck, and *Organic Manifesto*, by Maria Rodale. Each of these books is a wealth of information and well worth your time to read.

Holistic Medicine

About 95% of every healthcare dollar is
spent on treatment and less than 5% on prevention.
Holistic medicine espouses the prevention
of deadly diseases, type 2 diabetes,
coronary artery disease, stroke and colon cancer
by lifestyle choices, nutrition,
and supplemental herbs and spices.

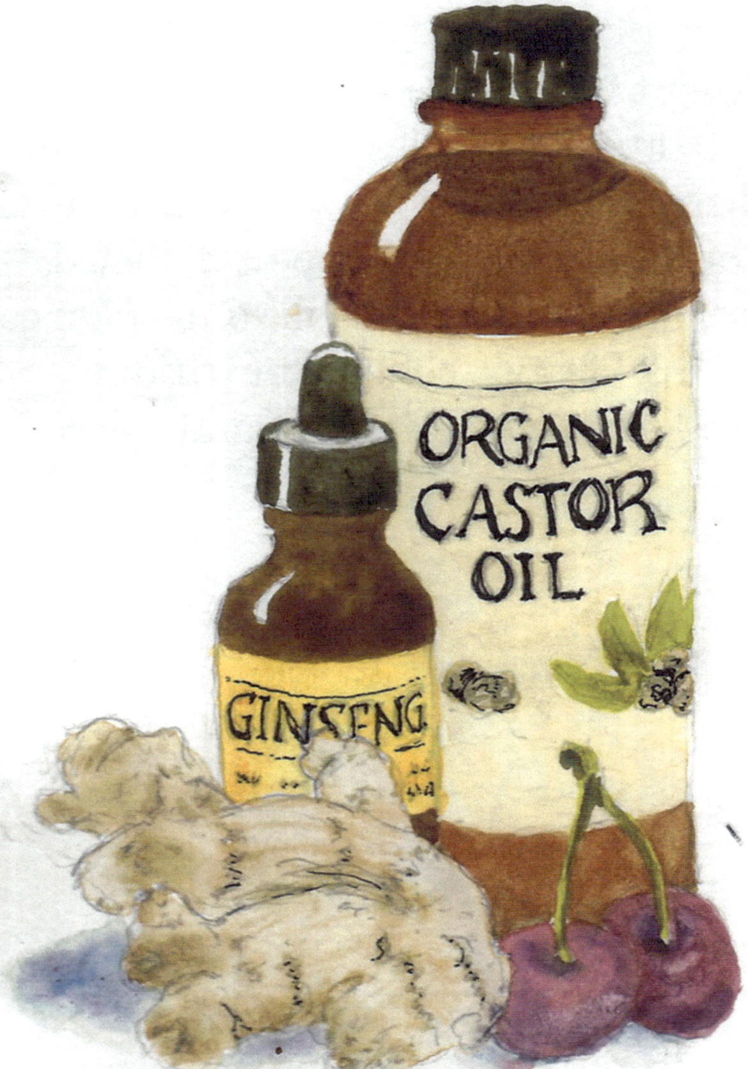
ORGANIC
CASTOR
OIL
GINSENG

The Amazing Castor Oil Pack

Edgar Cayce was an American psychic who allegedly possessed the ability to answer questions on healing while in a trance. While lying on a couch, with his wife reading him the name and address of whomever asked for help, he would give a solution. He lived from 1877 to 1945 in Virginia Beach, Virginia, and gave thousands of readings that are kept in the files of the A.R.E (Association for Research and Enlightenment). He is known as the "The Sleeping Prophet."

He popularized the use of cold-pressed castor oil in the 1940's and 50's and is the originator of the "Castor Oil Pack," which resulted in amazing health recoveries for many people. The use of castor oil Cayce most frequently recommended was as a castor oil pack. This is a square of unbleached white wool flannel, saturated with castor oil, applied to the abdomen, and covered by a plastic sheet. A heating pad covers it all, warming the area. It is good to use it for about three evenings at a time, for about an hour or an hour-and-a-half duration. I find it convenient and rewarding to use a pack every few months in the evening after getting ready for bed, and I read while using the pack.

Cayce recommended the use of castor oil packs in hundreds of readings to improve the body's eliminations, lymphatic circulation, and assimilation of nutrients. By using castor oil packs, the flow of lymph is increased throughout the body. This helps speed the removal of toxins surrounding the cells and reduce the size of swollen lymph nodes. The result is an improvement in organ function and a lessening of fatigue and depression. The results were so astounding that castor oil packs are still extremely popular today.

Dr. William McGarey, a Phoenix, Arizona, medical doctor, intensively studied Cayce's readings and applied them in his clinic. He recounts in his book, *The Oil that Heals*, that the castor oil packs were the key therapy for seemingly miraculous healings, helping his patients overcome disorders in a very short period of time. Castor oil appears to work by drawing blood circulation and enhanced biological energy to the area where it is applied, then drawing lodged toxins out of the body. Castor oil has proven very valuable in helping to detoxify the body at deeper levels, thus eliminating the root cause.

Ricinoleic Acid is effective in preventing the growth of numerous species of viruses, bacteria, yeasts, and molds. Castor oil is a triglyceride of fatty acids and almost 90% of its content consists of ricinoleic acid—thus it may be responsible for castor oil's remarkable healing abilities.

Because of its many beneficial effects, it can be applied topically to treat a wide variety of health complaints.

Castor oil has been used therapeutically for thousands of years in ancient China, Persia, Egypt, India, Africa, Greece, Rome, in 17th century Europe, and in the Americas. Castor oil was called the *Palma Christi*, or the" Hand of Christ" because of its healing properties. It is known to be effective for many diverse types of pain, liver and gallbladder cleansing and detoxing, digestive problems, eye irritations, lacerations, skin disorders such as eczema and psoriasis, ringworm, skin inflammation, constipation, menopause symptoms, keratoses, and much more. Castor oil enhances the immune system!

Cayce's recommendations for usage of castor oil were numerous for conditions such as cholecystitis (inflammation of the gallbladder), poor elimination, epilepsy, various liver conditions (cirrhosis and torpid liver), scleroderma, headaches, appendicitis, arthritis, colitis, colon impaction, nervous system coordination, and neuritis.

Joanne Boudreau, our 'Herb Lady' here in *Living Naturally First*, wrote that she uses gentle cleanses instead of harsh methods, and named Castor Oil Packs as a perfect product. As you can see, there are multiple uses and users.

I have found a small manufacturing company, Camelot Supply Company, that makes a Castor Oil Pack flannel that is more easily used than others, as it is a very thick wool flannel, measuring 10" by 14" wide. Most other castor oils packs on the market are made of much thinner wool flannel or cotton flannel material that has to be folded two or three times to make a pack that is thick enough for usage. But because Camelot's extra thick/single layer flannel material is thick enough to use without folding, it is easier to both apply and clean up after use than with most standard folded and multi-layered versions. It can be used many times and does not have to be tossed after using once. (If it has become rancid-smelling after a number of uses, then toss it.) I have used my Camelot Wool Flannel for several years now. It is the same cost as others, $10.95 plus tax and shipping. If you are interested, call me and I will be happy to send you one.

You can purchase your cold-pressed castor oil in a health food or drug store. It should be hexane free and contain no coloring, fragrance, or petroleum products. It is inexpensive and easy to find. Most families already have a heating pad. If not, you will have to purchase one. Then you will have the flannel, the castor oil, and the heating pad to make a castor oil pack.

(Editor's note: Camelot Supply Company is no longer in existence.)

April Fools! Simple Solutions

Even though it is "Aprils Fool" month, I'm not fooling when I give you these solutions for daily health problems. They work easily and safely, with no side-effects like drugs have.

When you fall, bump, or bruise yourself (not on cuts), rub a bit of Arnica salve on the hurt spot, and then place five little Arnica Montana pellets under your tongue until dissolved. The bruise will leave in a day or two, and you will be free of discomfort or pain. This builds new tissues. *Boiron* is the manufacturer. This product is homeopathic. I learned this when I ran after someone in the forest and tripped on a root and flew ten or fifteen feet. I put my hands out to stop my fall and really hurt my shoulder. Thinking I tore my rotator cuff, I called a nurse, and she told me to buy Arnica. It is inexpensive, too, costing about $11.00 for both the tube of pellets and tube of salve. Any drugstore carries Arnica.

If your husband develops gout (usually it is the man who gets gout), which is very painful, have him drink some black cherry juice, and it will leave. It is a good idea not eat mushrooms or organ meat if you are prone to gout. Gout is caused by uric acid, and one source is too much fructose, usually by drinking other fruit juices. Whole fruit is OK, because you are consuming fiber along with the fructose.

Again and again, the medical profession has warned us not to use salt, because it can raise our blood pressure and cause a heart attack. That is true about refined white salt, high in sodium chloride, which we have been consuming for years! But salt is good for us if *not* refined, and we need the iodine in our system. Buy sea salt. It is unrefined, and you should have a teaspoon each day for health. I buy Redmond's "Real Salt," which contains 53+ trace minerals and iodine.

(Editor's note: Another advantage of Redmond's Real Salt is the fact that it is mined from an ancient deposit that is pre-pollution.)

Other sea salt is good but look for iodine in the product. Dr. Steve Nelson of the Palm Desert's Synergy Wellness Clinic says he has actually lowered patients' blood pressure with sea salt and water (most people with high blood pressure are lacking enough water.)

Instead of using a sugar substitute such as Aspartame (Equal, NutraSweet) which causes brain damage; Splenda, which is a pesticide; Sucralose, which promotes bladder cancer… use Stevia, a healthy natural green leaf plant, or Xylitol, also healthy, which stops bacteria from creating cavities in your teeth and builds bone. Xylitol makes your teeth enamel so slick that the bacteria cannot climb up the tooth. There is a new spray form of Xylitol, too, called Xclear, that stops allergies, asthma, and sinus infections.

For motion/car sickness or nausea, chew some crystallized ginger. Ginger in your spice closet is one of the most effective antioxidants, along with cinnamon and turmeric. Cinnamon is a deterrent to blood sugar in diabetes. Turmeric (which is the yellow in mustard) is on top of the charts for immune system support. If you use three spices in each meal, it will promote health (pepper is a spice).

We have known for a long time that cranberry juice clears up bladder and urinary tract infections, but now we find out that it is a form of the simple sugar D-mannose, which is most effective against serious infections. Dr. Jonathon Wright said D-mannose has the ability to detach E-coli from the walls of the bladder without upsetting the balance of the friendly bacteria necessary for good health. After being loosened from bladder walls, the bacteria are rinsed away by normal urination. The E-coli are not killed; they're simply relocated—"from the inside to the outside"—and the infection is gone. One-half to one teaspoon taken in water every two to three hours, for two to three days, will eliminate almost any bladder infection caused by e-coli, and it has a great advantage of tasting incredibly good! Despite being classified as a "sugar," it is safe even for diabetics.

Elderberry juice concentrate, not elderberry cough syrup or other concentrations, helps promote healthy nasal, throat, and breathing passages. One or two teaspoons each morning does wonders. You can mix it with water for a drink or add it to whatever vegetables or fruits you have put through your juicer.

If you have problems with leg cramping, you may need magnesium. I take a 500 mg. capsule before bedtime, as it also aids in good sleep. You can buy magnesium oil and mix it one part oil to three parts water and spray it on your body. Our "Herb Lady," Jo Anne Boudreau, says to spray your children after their evening shower, and they will sleep better and do better in school the next day.

Other sleep aids are the amino acid, L-tryptophan, and the hormone, Melatonin, both safe and aid good moods. Doctors in *Breakthrough* said drug companies found a bogus reason to take L-tryptophan off the market a while back because it interfered with the sale of their drug, Prozac.

Colloidal Silver is a healing aid. It can be used in the mouth, eyes, nose, and ears, and you can drink it. Swimmers' ear is helped, mouth sores are banished, and the beginning of a cold or illness may benefit from its use early on.

Eating a serving of beans supplies nourishment, while helping to stop carbohydrates from forming fat around your middle. I lost three inches around my waist and stomach in two months by eating one serving of beans each day. There are enough varieties so you will not get tired of them. Beans are a starch neutralizer and are a healthy protein.

Instead of taking the drug, valium, anxiety can be stemmed by Kava-Kava, Gaba, or L-tryptophan with no side-effects.

Dr. Nelson said to buy a small trampoline and jump on it several times a day to move the lymph in your body. He said exercise and walking are great, but only jumping loosens the lymph (besides, you feel like a kid again, like you did with a jump-rope).

There are many other simple natural remedies. Do some reading and research and find them for yourself. It is so much easier to live with health, than to be talked into using drugs… WHICH HAVE SIDE EFFECTS YOU DO NOT WANT TO LIVE WITH!!

Earthing

Clint Ober, a cable television and computer marketer, had everything money could buy, when he developed a serious liver infection and almost died after painful and extensive surgery. A long mending process made him realize he had become a slave to his possessions, so he decided to set himself free and dedicate his life to something worthwhile, and with a purpose. He sold his business to his employees, sold his home, gave away any possessions his grown children did not want, and bought a recreational vehicle to drive the U.S.A, to find himself and his mission.

He became aware in his travels that everyone had on some kind of shoes or flip-flops, and no one was connected to the EARTH. He knew from his years in the cable industry that everything must be grounded. Could wearing rubber or plastic-lined shoes affect health by insulating us from the ground? His subsequent research found that we do have to be connected to Earth to be grounded… to receive Earth's energy.

This is called "EARTHING." It is a process of "grounding" ourselves by walking barefoot, connecting to Mother Earth. Grass, soil, stones, rock, and concrete that is not sealed or painted, all "ground" us… especially ocean sand. Asphalt, wood, plastic, bamboo, painted or sealed concrete do not work, as they do not allow electrons to pass through to your feet. Grounding counteracts the inflammation that causes disease in our bodies.

Inflammation Is the Primary Cause of Virtually All Disease. The surface of the Earth itself is one gigantic ANTI-inflammatory energizer, transferring healing *free electrons* into your body. Free radicals are what harm your immune system… and free electrons from the earth's surface counteract rampaging free radicals. There is a transfer of free electrons into your body through the soles of your feet! *The sole of the foot is covered with 1,300 nerve endings per square inch. (No other part of the body compares.)*

Our skin is a great conductor. The middle of the ball of the foot is known in acupuncture as "K-1" (Kidney One)… and it connects to all acupuncture meridians in the body. It essentially connects to every nook and cranny of your body. These electrons are some of the *most potent antioxidants* known to man!

Electrons come from the sun, to the ionosphere, to our earth. We function electrically on an electrical planet. We are a collection of dynamic electrical circuits. The earth beneath your feet contains great healing energy. Connection to earth establishes normal rhythms for repair, recovery, rejuvenation. Disconnection sets up the immune system for malfunction, an electron deficiency. Electron deficiency is from loss of direct contact with earth. It is called "electro-pollution"!!! The electron contacts are slowed down or totally missing. As a result, an increase in chronic illness has become quite evident.

As a society, we are hurting and unhealthy. We are disconnected from earth, our homes are plasticized and insulated; insulation that is stopping our connection to earth from our homes, offices, and other buildings, creating unnecessary suffering in the form of inflammation, sickness, pain, and poor sleep. Connecting to the earth is the simple solution to remedy that deficiency. Grounding powerfully reduces the inflammation that causes the illness by counteracting electromagnetic fields (emf) in your body. Earthing is revolutionary, a discovery of the first magnitude, as potentially significant and globally sweeping as were electricity, automobiles, telephones, radio, television, cell phones, computers, and the Internet. Earthing can change the way medicine is practiced, adding major effectiveness in healing and lowering the cost of treatment.

There was a great deal of skepticism from the medical establishment. They needed everything double-blind tested in the lab. Clint Ober did his own testing and research by using a system of electric tape connected by a wire to an outside grounding rod. He formed electric patches, the same kind used by doctors when they do EKG (electrocardiogram) tests. His subjects' pain left them, and they called his patches "Magic Pain Patches." He added the electric wire to pads and then sheets, and those that slept on them stopped having insomnia and other physical problems. He tried the sheets on sixty women he found in beauty shops who could not sleep well. The majority of them lessened or ceased their insomnia. He found his grounding materials helped all kinds of physical problems.

After four or five years of practicing on all kinds of volunteers, he convinced a biophysicist, Dr. James Oschman, who has now become the top energy medicine expert, to test his discovery. Dr. Oschman took "Earthing" into the laboratory so it would be believable to the medical profession. He used thermal photographic images in his clinic to discern the effects. He used infrared imaging. He took a picture of a man's body, then had him walk on the ground for thirty minutes, then took another picture. All of the tissue damage revealing red inflammation on the first picture now showed lack of inflammation in blue and green imaging on the second picture. They illustrated a rapid resolution of pain and stiffness.

He used thermal imaging on long-term open wounds and found healing and improvement in circulation. Treatment of daily thirty-minute grounding sessions healed a woman's wound after she had undergone treatments in a specialized wound center for eight months with no results.

There has been success in many different circumstances. People who sleep grounded are calmer, more energetic, and less stressed during the day, waking up with less stiffness and soreness in the morning; people with asthma and respiratory ailments, such as bronchitis and emphysema, breathe better; headaches often become less intense and frequent and sometimes go away altogether; heartburn and acid reflux benefit from grounding after walking for twenty minutes; grounding may make constipation go away; earthing helps circulation; eczema and psoriasis improve; dry skin and dry itchy eyes improve; for bedridden individuals, a grounded bed sheet can reduce or eliminate bedsores.

Jeff Spencer, who is the doctor for the Tour de France cyclists, uses overnight grounding for accelerated wound healing when his cyclists skid and fall.

Clint has now developed Earthing Shoes, Earthing Pads for the floor that can be used by putting bare feet on them when using the computer, or under the mouse with your arm resting on it: Earthing Sheets for the bed; Earthing Sleeping Bags; Earthing Body and Knee bands: Earthing Patches; Earthing beds and even Earthing Pet Pads. You can look them up on the Internet at earthinginstitute.net and order them at earthing.com.

I always try whatever I find that heals, and I bought a sheet and patches, and they solved my sleeping problem and back pain from an auto accident.

I then called my brother. He called two men whom he knew had illnesses. The first, eighty-five years old, had been well until eight months before. Ten days later, he called and said that after walking outside for thirty minutes, four times a day, he was now well. The second, eighty years old, was wealthy and had knee pain for years, even after exhaustive medical attention and physical therapy. He bought a sheet and called my brother to tell him that after the second night, his knee pain was gone. After three nights the IBS (Irritable Bowel Syndrome) he had for nine months with diarrhea and constipation was gone. And sinus problems he had for a long time left after the third morning, when he sneezed everything out, and it was gone. His sleeping routine had also changed, and he now awoke full of energy.

I knew this from Clint Ober's book, *Earthing*, that he solved problems like these:

- A woman with five years of debilitating pain, inflammation, sleep problems, and fatigue after a serious car accident had gone from one practitioner to another, with no change, slept on this sheet. In a few months, all her problems vanished.
- After a long air trip, one woman arrived at her destination jet-lagged, and after she took her shoes off and walked outside for thirty minutes, it stopped.
- A man, so badly arthritic it took others to lift him out of bed, complained a week later that a squirrel had chewed the grounding wire outside. When Ober checked, the man was standing in his doorway, watching.
- A woman with crippling arthritis was in such severe pain that she could not even hold the handheld tester. Ten minutes after the electrode patch was put on her arm, she asked that it be put on the other arm because the pain level had improved so considerably.
- Men described having better erections and experiencing fewer trips to urinate at night, as a result of sleeping grounded.

I know that all of this seems amazing, but you cannot really grasp the depth of this until you pick up *Earthing* and read it yourself. I cannot express what you will achieve after reading it.

Hormonal Therapy Is A Necessity

Dr. Thierry Hertogue, the Father of Bio-Identicals in Europe, stated, *"Hormones are crucial to every single function of the human body. You can't live without them!"* Today, through cutting-edge, alternative medicine, our knowledge now states… Hormone Replacement is restoration! Restoration stops deterioration and aging! REPLACE HORMONES THAT HAVE BEEN LOST AND GET YOUR YOUTH BACK!

But many of us have a bad remembrance of the debacle of synthetic Hormone Replacement Therapy of the 1970's. After three decades, a study was made. It was stopped in 2002, when test results showed it caused increased risk of invasive breast cancer, heart disease, stroke, and blood clots in lungs (pulmonary congestion).

Hormone Replacement Therapy consisted mainly of Provera, Prempro, or Premarin, (pregnant mare's urine... a mare is put in a stall for life, with a catheter in her bladder to extract the urine and is impregnated for fifteen years until she dies.)

Dr. Khalid Mahmud, who for twenty-five years was a very successful oncologist here in the U.S., wasn't happy with the western model for disease care and switched to an anti-aging alternative preventive practice. He found pharmaceutical corporations produced these synthetic hormones because they could patent them. They were expensive... and the industry is built on profit, lots of profit!

Six years ago (*Editor's note: 2009) he said, "66% of all department chairs at universities in America have financial contracts with pharmaceutical corporations. Our medical schools are compromised because they *can't teach* about natural remedies or natural hormones or they will lose their financial grants.

This is shocking; this means pharmaceutical companies are in control of our universities, our government officials, our airwaves, and our print media. When I start patients on bio-identical hormones, they then go to their regular doctors, who tell them not to take them, because there are no studies. There have been many positive studies in Europe for fifty or sixty years. We know the answer: bio-identical hormones are not patentable, and businesses are not interested in promoting a drug, no matter how beneficial, if they can't own the patent."

The answer is *Bio-Identical Hormones*:

Estrogen is very important for memory and multi-tasking. It acts in the brain to make connections in the hypothalamus and memory sensors. It repairs damage to nerve cells, and fights beta peptides which cause Alzheimer's.

Testosterone improves overall muscle tone, makes muscles tighter (you can work with a trainer all day, but without testosterone, you can't get anywhere), builds bone, provides good sex drive, improves energy, enhances brain function, decreases body fat, creates good hand-eye coordination and competitiveness, gives a sense of security. Since the heart is the largest muscle in the body, testosterone is an important hormone for the heart, decreasing inflammation, protecting the heart.

Testosterone is produced in the ovaries and testes. It improves clitoral and nipple sensitivity, increases libido, improves the quality of orgasm, increases muscle strength and bone density, and provides a good mood.

DHEA is the Mother Hormone. It is made in our brain and our adrenal cortex. It increases testosterone, muscle mass, decreases body fat, improves memory, decreases depression, improves our immune system, lowers cholesterol and insulin levels. It also helps prevent a decrease in mental function as a precursor to Parkinson's or Alzheimer's diseases, since it protects neurons in our brain.

Progesterone is the balance. Dr. John Lee is the original doctor who brought *natural progesterone* into the limelight, counteracting the harmful synthetic "progestin" that was prevalent in the hormone replacement therapy of the 1970's and 1980's. In 1978, Dr. Lee learned of natural progesterone made from plants by Dr. Ray Peet. At the time, when women started menopause, or had a hysterectomy, doctors gave unopposed estrogen. But Dr. Lee knew "Mother Nature" has always arranged for estrogen and progesterone to be made at the same time. He thought, "The ovary makes two hormones… why aren't we giving two hormones?"

Estrogen, after menopause, only drops 40% to 50% even though the ovaries are no longer producing, but Dr. Lee realized doctors were not aware of this and gave two, four, or eight times too much estrogen, thinking the lack was the problem. Fat women produce more estrogen than thin women, since estrogen is produced through fat cells after menopause.

Dr. Lee then started giving many patients progesterone cream for one year, using no estrogen. They began to lose the swollen breasts, fibrocystic breasts, fat around the middle and hips and abdomen, depression, foot swelling from sitting too long, water retention… and gained back their interest in sex, and their bones got better.

He reversed osteoporosis with progesterone. He found a deficiency of progesterone was a common malady long before menopause.

Progesterone is necessary to make the myelin sheath. The myelin sheath protects and covers all the nerves as they pass through your body. These little cells make a covering, an insulation called myelin that protects the nerve, so it does not short-circuit and lose its electric impulse.

The body is complex. This hormone does so many things. Brain cells concentrate progesterone and testosterone twenty times higher than the blood carries. Dr. Lee understood why patients who gave progesterone to their mothers or aged aunts in nursing homes for their bones and to hydrate their skin caused them to become more alert and aware. When they had been content to lie in bed all day and could not keep track of conversation… after a week or so of being on progesterone, they were up leading discussion of the headlines.

A doctor from Sao Paulo, Brazil, gave it to his ninety-two-year-old mother, who resumed being an intellectual giant again, where before, she had become a baby-like cripple. (This doctor now specializes in the care of the elderly.)

People think they understand progesterone, but they are ignorant of the fact that progesterone is involved throughout the body, from the nerves to the brain cells, to the thyroid gland, to fat metabolism, to muscle building energy.

Progesterone is absorbed by rubbing it on the skin… forty to seventy times more efficient than swallowing by mouth. (Being fat soluble, it goes to the liver and then to the bile. Only 5% gets through and puts the liver to work.)

Progesterone does not show in a blood test, because it goes to the fat cells. The saliva gland tells how much progesterone you have. There is a simple saliva test. Go to a compounding pharmacy and ask for a saliva test. They will send off your vial and the correct amount of estrogen, progesterone, testosterone, and DHEA will be prescribed, which the pharmacy will then compound for you each month.

What Doctor John Lee has told us is that balanced bio-identical hormones are crucial, and we are fools if we think we don't need them after menopause. All the old ladies you see in nursing homes with thin bones, memory loss, no energy… just existing… are mainly there from a lack of hormones since menopause. The percentage of women using hormones past menopause is very small.

We have to change this outlook with education of our women.

Bio-identical hormones are our solution. Normalize your hormones and your life!

Naturopathic vs. Conventional Medicine

Life Extension magazine is a very refreshing spokesman for preventative and holistic medicine and has been published for many years. This month, they are opening a glimpse into the fact that there has been controversy between allopathic (conventional) medicine backed by the American Medical Association and big pharmaceutical corporations, and functional medicine in the form of Naturopathic, Holistic, Herbal, and Alternative medicine for over a hundred years... but conventional medicine's house of cards is about to begin its big fall from grace with the recent announcement that the prestigious Cleveland Clinic is going "functional."

President and CEO of the Cleveland Clinic, Dr. Delos "Toby" Cosgrove, announced a number of significant actions: Establishment of the first functional medicine grand rounds entitled "Functional Perspective on Food and Nutrition: The Ultimate Upstream Medicine." Included are:

- Research to test functional medicine models head-to-head against conventional medicine for a number of chronic diseases, such as diabetes, asthma, and autoimmune diseases.
- The creation of a Wellness Institute and the appointment of the nation's first Chief Wellness Officer.
- Creation of a Chinese Herbal Therapy Clinic, one of the first of its kind in the country.
- The movement of the clinic's $6.2 billion network of hospitals, family health centers, and outpatient clinics in a decidedly holistic direction.

The money-driven medical establishment has been able to hold off this trend with some clever political spin tactics. They have consistently attacked Natural Medicine using orthodox medical associations while "Big Pharma" uses its enormous wealth to control Congress, large numbers of medical schools and the media. They have put forth such a constantly heavy marketing campaign that We, the Public, have been brainwashed... for years!

Conventional medicine has been acquiring a very dismal track record on the treatment of chronic disease. Negative developments occurring regarding conventional medicine include:

- The GDP of health care expenditures is increasing…from 5.2% in 1960 and estimated to reach nearly 20% by 2021.
- The U.S. spends nearly twice as much as other industrialized countries on healthcare per capita but ranks near the bottom in almost every measure of our population health.
- About 95% of every healthcare dollar is spent on treatment and less than 5% on prevention. Holistic medicine espouses the prevention of deadly diseases, type 2 diabetes, coronary artery disease, stroke, and colon cancer by lifestyle choices, nutrition, and supplemental herbs and spices.
- *The New England Journal of Medicine* reported that over $100 billion was spent on balloon angioplasty and coronary artery bypass grafting in 2007, yet only 3% of bypass patients experienced prolonged life span.
- Prescription drugs cause 700,000 emergency room visits each year and over 41,000 deaths.
- Recent evidence estimates there are over 400,000 avoidable hospital deaths each year.

Dr. David Eddy did a study on the scientific evidence behind conventional medical treatments. *Business Week* magazine quoted Dr. Eddy's study in 2006 and declared that only 20% to 25% of what was done to treat patients has been proven effective.

There is still a problem related to the number of unnecessary operations being performed, such as knee surgery, back surgery, angioplasty, and heart surgery. Holistic medicine has other methods of coping with these illnesses.

In the late 1940's and early 1950's, Natural medicine pushed back. Nobel Laureate Linus Pauling led a small group of scientists and doctors to treat brain-related illnesses, such as depression and schizophrenia, with diet and nutritional supplements. The results of this new approach were pleasing and named the protocols as "orthomolecular psychiatry."

A hippy groundswell of the 1960's created interest in nonconventional treatments for the whole human body. Visits to naturopaths, chiropractors, and acupuncturists increased, while reports of dangerous side effects from prescription medications continued to surface.

In 1978, Joseph Pizzorno, co-founded Bastyr University in Portland, Oregon, to educate naturopathic doctors. It is now recognized as one of the premier schools in the world for natural medicine. We now have 1,800 naturopathic/holistic doctors in our country.

With the help of Senator Orrin Hatch of Utah, legislation passed under this title: "Dietary Supplement Health and Education Act of 1994" (DSHEA). It is a major law, and "Big Pharma" and the medical establishment keep trying to take the protection of dietary supplements away, since supplements have become a big business, and they are losing ground.

Conventional doctors have been trained to look for specific symptoms and treat them with pharmaceutical drugs or surgery. Naturopathic doctors consider the whole body, use prevention first, and then promote correct food, supplements, and exercise to heal the body.

Since World War II, food processing has made a major change in our "REAL FOOD" to substitute many synthetic, harmful, addictive substances to its packages, bottles, cans, and bags, altering the health of our nation. We do not consume enough vitamins, minerals, amino acids, and enzymes in the majority of our processed food to supply our needs, thus the need for supplements.

Our soil has been compromised by synthetic fertilizers, pesticides, and insecticides for the same amount of time, and there is rarely enough nutrition in the plants being grown. The best chance of fulfilling our needs is to purchase our food in farmer's markets, where most of the produce is organic, and most of the meats—chicken, beef, bison, lamb, and goat—are grass-fed and finished (not put into feed lots for the last eight months of their lives… and fed corn, given antibiotics and growth hormones, and sprayed with pesticides). Processed food has coined the word "Natural" for product packaging because the public connects that with "Healthy."

Natural does not mean Organic!!! Once again, it is just done to attract sales.

Keep your eyes open. Read what is on the back of each package of food you buy. Look up:

American College for Advancement in Medicine… www.acam.org
National Foundation of Alternative Medicine… www.nfam.org
American Holistic Medical Association… www.Holisticmedicine.org.

Enter your zip code and find a Naturopathic Doctor near you.

(Editor's Note: this paper was published in June 2015.)

No More Drilling! Stop and Reverse Dental Decay

As I delve further into research, finding methods of how to stay well, how to build up the immune system, how to avoid illness and disease by natural means instead of by drugs and/or surgery, I am constantly outraged at how much information has been hidden from us. When I stumble upon one miraculous, simple method after another, of preventing or healing painful, expensive disease… each breakthrough reinforces the knowledge of how much is out there that we are blind to, knowledge that would amaze and anger us to realize we do not have to go through pain, fear, worry, and monetary depletion to "fix" the problem.

Don't you wonder, as I do, why this information is being kept quiet? Who gains from our pain? Who sweeps it under the carpet?

My daughter, who like me, is in good health and rarely has a health problem, had been sorely aching from a dental procedure, and after two weeks asked for a second opinion. Since the second dentist could not give her an answer, except that the x-ray seemed to show a gray area with possibly some extra hidden bacteria, I decided to look into the subject.

Once again, I found a simply amazing procedure that has been in practice for ninety years in Cuba, fifty years in Russia, and as recently as 2002, *in every country except the United States*.

Dr. Julian Holmes of the UK says we were not availed of this procedure because the FDA did not approve of the delivery machinery. This *new* technology is Ozone Air Abrasion.

There is no drilling the tooth to eliminate the cavity bacteria and then filling the tooth to close it. A small rubber nozzle aims ozone into the area, and all the bacteria and decay are cleared out and sterilized. It does not destroy tooth tissue to eliminate the bacteria. Just a sixty-second burst of ozone will destroy all the bacteria that caused the infection and decay.

Damage to the tooth is limited, with no need to amputate a large volume of tooth structure. By effectively sterilizing the lesion, minerals from the patient's own saliva will re-enter the area, re-mineralize, and harden them. Once hardened, it is more resistant to future bacterial attack and mineral loss.

Dr. Holmes says, "Every dentist is trained to drill the decay out or amputate it and then replace it with a filling. There is no going back. Each time the filling needs to be removed and replaced, there is little left of the original tooth and a larger filling is required each subsequent time."

I looked on the Internet and found a dentist close to us. He took care of my daughter's pain and used the Ozone abrasion. He told us that it takes three months for the bacteria to return. It only takes four to six weeks for our saliva to re-mineralize the holes the decay left. If we wanted, he had some form of material he could spray on the tooth for immediate coverage.

In fact, he had a little six-year-old boy in his chair with a bad cavity, and in thirty minutes or less, the little boy walked out with his mother, with his tooth healed, and smiling instead of frightened and crying. It is the only time I have ever seen patients smiling and hugging dentists and nurses in a reception room.

The dentist told us this is possible now, thanks to a major innovation that has been developed over the last twenty years in Europe, Canada, Africa, and South America. It's called Ozone Technology or Activated Oxygen. Ozone is known to have a remarkable ability to both kill bad bacteria as well as kick-start our healing process. Ozone is the same material used microscopically at a cellular level by our body to get rid of infection.

Most human cells are immune to ozone, but the activated form of oxygen kills all known germs, bacteria, fungi, and viruses without harming our own cells.

Ozone has also proved very useful in stopping annoying cold sore outbreaks and to desensitize painful teeth and remove canker sores inside the mouth. Only a small handful of dentists have studied this technology in the U.S., although many other professionals have been using ozone for years outside the country with great success.

The Internet sites I found were under Ozone Dentistry, Ozone Therapy, Laser Dentistry.

Find a dentist near you and stop hurting.

Oriental Medicine Tidbits

I get a variety of mail from doctors and healing resources of all kinds. I believe my name has been sold to anyone who wants to peddle to me natural methods of improving our health and immunity. My mailbox is overflowing… so much so that I am now calling each of these contacts to take my name off their mailing lists. (The Post Office will make me buy a postal box ten times the size I have now.) Some of the information is factual and interesting enough for me to research. I decided to give my readers the interesting tidbits I have culled from all the myriads of letters, brochures, magazines, etc.

From Eastern and Chinese medicine:

A tri-herb combination of licorice, ginseng, and glechoma (a flowering plant) was given to fifty-five patients with hypothyroidism in a study published in *Natural Journal of Medicine Forum*. Fifty-three of them improved—an eye-popping 97% success rate. Good luck finding a thyroid drug with that kind of success!

U.S. cancer researchers have found that ginger kills ovarian cancer cells *in vitro*. Miraculously, ginger causes two types of death to cancer cells: apoptosis (the usual kind) and autophagy (where one cancer cell attacks another).

The ancient herb that clears arteries like "Drano" …gingko biloba contains "flavonoids" which are plant-derived antioxidants that help clear arteries and make blood vessel functions strong. A new study published in *Circulation* shows it lowers the risk of peripheral artery disease.

Reported in *Phytomedicine*: green tea is even effective in protecting the brain from hydrogen peroxide and beta amyloids—toxins that cause Alzheimer's.

"Palm" your eyes! Rub your hands together, then cover your closed eyes with the palms of your hands. This promotes extreme relaxation, relaxes tense eyeballs, and relieves strain –all for clear, pinpoint vision.

"Viagra" has a 73% success rate for erectile dysfunction, but the listed side effects may include blurry vision, upset stomach, headaches, diarrhea, dizziness—and in rare cases, prolonged erections. In a study reported in the *Journal of Applied Traditional Chinese Medicine*, a 94% success rate, with no side effects, was found from "Jiao Tai," a natural pill made of seven herbs well-known among Chinese herbalists for treating erectile dysfunction.

Chinese Masters believe pain is often the result of blockages in your body's energy flow (known as Qi and pronounced 'chi'). But you can undo these blockages with simple massages known as acupressure—the first cousin of acupuncture, but with no needles. One secret prized by Chinese doctors for knee pain is the "Reducing Technique."

Simply find the special "acupoint ST35" right below your knee, in the little pocket to the outside of your kneecap. By putting firm pressure with your thumb and middle finger—and massaging in a clockwise manner for two to three minutes—you can make knee pain vanish, almost instantly.

Chronic Fatigue affects women two to four times as often as men… sore throats, chronic coughs, mystery aches and pains, anxiety, headaches, and weariness are the complaints. Western doctors prescribe drugs. The Center for Disease Control lists these drugs as anti-depressants, NSAIDS, tricyclic agents, anxiety agents, anti-microbials and anti-allergy medications.

Chinese medicine sees Chronic Fatigue as a disruption of your body's energy flow. Their solution is "Bu Zhong Yi Qi Tang," a unique mix of eight herbs including licorice, citrus, and astragalus. 80% of patients improved, as opposed to 32% using drugs.

❦ ❦ ❦

Traditional Chinese medicine tells patients suffering from pain, insomnia, memory loss, or physical weakness to walk on cobblestones. This secret is rooted in the ancient belief of "reflexology." The uneven surface of the cobblestones stimulates the soles of the feet and triggers acupoints. American researchers visiting China saw adults spending a half-hour every day on cobblestone paths in parks, gardens, and riverbanks. In a National Institute of Aging study, it was found that doing this three times a week for four months had huge reductions in blood pressure, as well as improvements in balance and physical performance.

My sources say, "If Western medicine's 'CUT, BURN, AND MEDICATE' treatments are not working for you or causing harmful side effects, find a 'Master of Chinese Medicine'."

Prolotherapy: Knee Cartilage Healing

While doing research for my columns and seminars on natural healing, I frequently come across an exciting nonsurgical, non-pharmaceutical solution to a common problem. Many people have knees that exhibit torn or lost cartilage—from sports injuries, arthritis, accidents, or from wear and tear, or age—and are told they need a knee replacement. This entails surgery, several painful months of therapy, and a great deal of expense.

Susan, one of my clients who happens to be a pharmacist, experienced a new way to build back the cartilage without surgery, at one-tenth the cost. It is known as Prolotherapy, or Regenerative Injection Therapy, a medical procedure that involves the injection of natural substances into weakened musculoskeletal tissue to stimulate repair. This is a permanent treatment. I contacted her kind and patient orthopedic doctor in Austin, Dr. Bradley Fullerton, who spent an hour explaining the process.

A solution is injected into the knee, which irritates the joint and causes inflammation.

The inflammation causes your immune system to send healing cells to the area to repair the damage.

- Your body sends more blood to the area, delivering oxygen and nutrients.
- Immune cells called *macrophages* remove debris from the area.

Next, your immune system sends *fibroblasts*, which are the cells that make new cartilage. This happens naturally in your body every day, making it possible to heal injuries that the body can't heal on its own. This procedure also heals back joints and hips.

Another doctor who practices this prolotherapy is Frank Shallenberger, who sends out a health newsletter each month and has several books available. He noticed that younger patients got much better results from the treatment than older ones. A leading cause of aging is the inability to get oxygen into the cells. The *New England Journal of Medicine* concluded that the single biggest difference between a twenty-five-year-old and a seventy-year-old is the utilization of oxygen. Doctor Shallenberger uses *ozone therapy*.

He makes sure the patient takes glucosamine and MSM (methysulfonylmethane, an essential sulfur nutrient, which helps heal connective tissue, aids in relieving pain, repairs damaged skin by circulating the production of collagen and increases blood circulation) the entire time he's seeing him. He also injects some cartilage-building nutrients directly into the joint, including vitamin B12 and hyaluronic acid (the major ingredient in joint fluid is hyaluronic acid). He first injects Novocain, then switches syringes and adds the prolotherapy solution, then unscrews that syringe and attaches a tube containing ozone. He says that the whole treatment takes about three minutes.

Despite the amazing success of this therapy, the conventional medical establishment continues to ignore it. New treatments are usually around for decades before the mainstream accepts them. A number of cutting-edge doctors are aware of the therapy and administer it. Over 90% of these patients leave with their cartilage back and their pain and inflammation gone.

Dr. Shallenberger has been teaching doctors how to use it for the past fifteen years. So far, well over 500 doctors around the world are using it. He teaches the use of *Prozolone*, his ozone therapy.

You can check out www.oygenhealingtherapies.com and check under Ozone therapy. Some doctors in Texas who use this therapy are:

- Dr. Barry Beatty, Ft. Worth, 817-737-6464
- Dr. William Coleman, Waco, 254-772-5353
- Dr. Kam Friedrichs, DC, Navasota, 936-825-6365
- Dr. Constantine Kotsanis, Grapevine, 817-481-6342
- Dr. Richard Massey, Fredericksburg, 830-990-2924
- Dr. Ron Manzanero, Austin, 512-343-6223
- Dr. James Paul, Houston, 281-894-1361

Secret Easy Fixes for Our Complicated, Modern, Chemical World

Today, with thousands of pharmaceutical drugs in conventional doctors' hands and mainstream medicine in control… backed by the government, we have forgotten the simple natural ways of our country doctors of old to heal and give succor. Today's cutting-edge doctors have not only *not forgotten* cures of the past, but have added new true technology, cures without drugs or surgery.

As I learn of each new breakthrough discovery, I am amazed and comforted to realize that the "Father of Medicine," Hippocrates, showed a great deal of forethought and knowledge when he said, "First, do no harm."

In the 1940's, penicillin was created to heal pneumonia, which at the time was almost a death warrant. And, in the 1950's with the polio epidemic killing and paralyzing us, Jonas Salk developed the Salk vaccine (because his wife contracted poliomyelitis, and he needed a cure for her). In the ensuing years, many drugs and vaccines have been developed that, instead of healing, have harmed the public. Our government has not done more than give a wrist-slap for truly detrimental drugs, developed in greed, bringing in billions of $$$, and were not consistently double-blind tested.

I will note this month some of the simple, amazing discoveries that have been cited by the cutting edge, alternative, anti-aging doctors whom I have researched. Some of the processes I enumerate are *new* technology; some are what we've all called "Grandma's Remedies."

From Dr. Julian Whitaker, Newport Beach, California Wellness Institute: Cover open wounds with sugar and change dressings every four to six days, a discovery in the 1980's by Dr. Richard Knutson of Greenville, Mississippi in *Medical World News*, who has treated over 7,000 patients successfully. Debridement, or removal of dead and infected tissue, is completely unnecessary because sugar stimulates natural debridement and promotes healing. Antibiotics are unwarranted, since no antibiotic comes close to sugar for local infection control, creating an environment in which no bacteria can survive. Sugar reduces edema and stimulates the growth of tissue to form new skin cells to cover and repair the lesion.

To treat any open wound, burn, laceration, scrape, or ulcer: mix a couple of tablespoons of white sugar with enough glycerin to form a peanut butter-like consistency. Open a 4" x 4" piece of gauze into a long strip, coat it with Vaseline, and place it around the wound. Put a thick layer of sugar/glycerin paste over the wound and cover with a sponge gauze. Secure with a cling dressing that holds the sugar in place but does not constrict. Change the dressing every four to six days by removing the gauze, rinsing the wound with water, saline, or hydrogen peroxide, drying it, and applying fresh sugar/glycerin.

Raw manuka honey may be used instead of sugar.

A second method of wound healing is to use hyperbaric oxygen therapy (HBOT). It must be done in a doctor's office, in a chamber that is slowly pressurized while you breathe 100% oxygen. Concentrated oxygen creates an inhospitable environment for most types of bacteria and prevents the spread of infection and speeds recovery from burns, bites, post-surgical incisions, bedsores, and sports injuries. Neither of these therapies is on the radar of most conventional doctors.

Gout is a very painful swelling caused by uric acid, a malady often linked to diabetes, and mostly to men. Instead of going to the doctor for shots in the joint or prescribing drugs, surprisingly, black cherry juice usually remedies this. Also, it is advisable to stay away from mushrooms and organ meats. Fructose promotes gout, so don't drink fruit juices which are pure fructose (other than black cherry)… if you do want fruit, eat the whole fruit, which has fiber. I offer my clients also a mineral supplement, KM, developed by Austrian Dr. Karl Jurak in the 1920's, that has also been a remedy.

Arnica relieves muscle pain and stiffness due to minor injuries, over-exertion, and falls. It reduces pain, swelling, and discoloration from bruises. Massage a thin layer of Arnica gel or cream to the affected area as soon as possible after injury. Put three to five tiny Arnica pellets under your tongue and dissolve. (The hardest part is not eating the pellets since they taste like candy.) Do this three times a day for several days. This is a very inexpensive procedure; the gel costs about $6.00 and the pellet tube about $5.00. I keep one set in my bathroom cabinet and one set in my car's glove compartment.

Our "Herb Lady," Jo Anne Boudreau, says that elderberry juice concentrate dries excess mucus in the sinuses, throat, lungs, stomach, and intestines. A teaspoon every morning also treats colds and flu, along with allergies and the respiratory system, and helps balance blood sugar.

Transdermal Magnesium oil spray has so many properties to heal us that it seems like a magic potion. A magnesium deficiency is on a grand scale here in the good ole' U.S.A. It accounts for depression, irritability, inability to deflect anger, irregular heartbeat, sleep disorders, numbness, hyperventilation, migraines, muscle cramps, obesity, and ADHD.

I take a 500 mg. magnesium citrate vitamin pill before bedtime, as it makes for a good night's sleep and completes my daily magnesium requirement. Jo Anne Boudreau says if you have chigger bites, spray them to dry them up. For toenail fungus, soak in two cups of water and one ounce of oil. Do this for several days in a row. Spray your children with this oil after their bedtime bath and they will sleep better and do well in school.

Edgar Cayce was known as the "Sleeping Prophet." He had only a grade school education, but could lie on the sofa, go into a trance, and give readings on healing, given a patient's name and location. He lived in Virginia Beach, Virginia, and there is an Edgar Cayce Foundation there with thousands of files of successful healings.

One of his main theses is the Castor Oil Pack. It is a wool flannel fabric that is doused with pure cold-pressed castor oil, placed on the abdomen, then covered with a heating pad for an hour or two. It rejuvenates the inner organs, breaks up and empties the toxins in the liver, gall bladder and intestines, and promotes healthy tissue. Sore spots and hurts on the body heal with this application for several days.

Dr. William A McGarey wrote the book, *The Oil That Heals*, and he and his wife, Dr. Gladys McGarey pioneered the treatment concepts found in the Edgar Cayce Readings. A second book, *The Miracle Oil*, by David Kukor has many case histories of practical castor oil applications.

I found the best source for the pack at Camelot Supply Company, but unfortunately, they have since closed. Drug stores sell cold pressed castor oil for about $10. It may be used over and over several times. This is a very inexpensive and easy process. You will want to put a plastic bag between the oil-soaked flannel and heating pad, as the oil is very tenacious.

Colloidal Silver is probably the most universal natural antibiotic substance. It is tasteless, non-addictive and nontoxic. Bacteria, fungus, and viruses do not seem to develop immunity to silver as they do to chemical antibiotic agents. Colloidal Silver will heal sores, blisters or cuts in the mouth, eye infections, ear infections, cold and flu viruses, shingles, and many more problems. Not for pregnant or nursing women.

Crystalized ginger aids car or plane nausea, inner ear nausea, tastes great, and is an effective agent for building immunity. Ginger, cinnamon, and turmeric are all great immunity builders. In fact, if you add three spices (pepper is a spice, salt is not) or herbs to each meal, you will greatly enhance your health. Cinnamon is a great blood sugar stabilizer. Putting a clove into the area of a toothache will ease the pain.

Tryptophan at bedtime will give you a good night's sleep and lift your mood. Tryptophan competed so well with Prozac for depressive moods, that the pharmaceutical giants saw to its removal from the market for years. It has been put back in the supplement market in the past several years. When it was taken off the market, I bought mine from veterinarians, who gave it to their animals.

We women knew that cranberry juice would stop bladder infections, but Dr. Jonathan Wright of the Tahoma Clinic in Washington state says the best cure is D-Mannose. The e-coli like sweetness, and they let go of the bladder walls and grab onto D-Mannose and are washed out along with it. Nontoxic.

You are aware of how wonderful coconut oil is, if you have read my columns, but I want to add that coconut oil is not only moisturizing to our skin, but it acts as a sunscreen that doesn't block the pores like commercial sunscreens do.

I teach Natural Health Nutrition seminars twice a month here in the Hill Country. If you are interested in living in vibrant health instead of disease and illness, come and open your eyes to a whole new, easy way of life with vitality, energy, sexuality, happiness… rejuvenate your life.

Health and Nutrition

Contrary to what you've heard,
cholesterol is NOT the cause of heart disease,
but rather a potent antioxidant weapon protecting
us against free radicals in the blood
that lead to heart disease.
Naturally produced in the body and naturally
present in the foods we eat, it is a repair substance
that actually helps heal arterial damage.

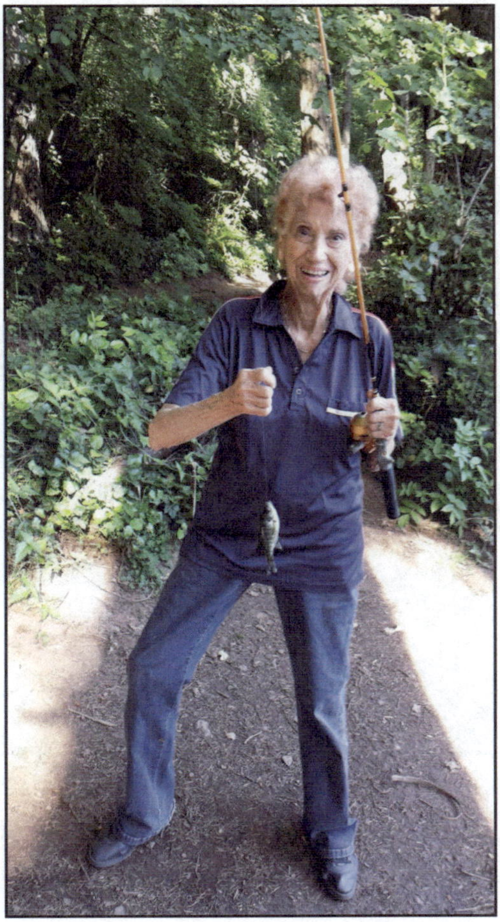

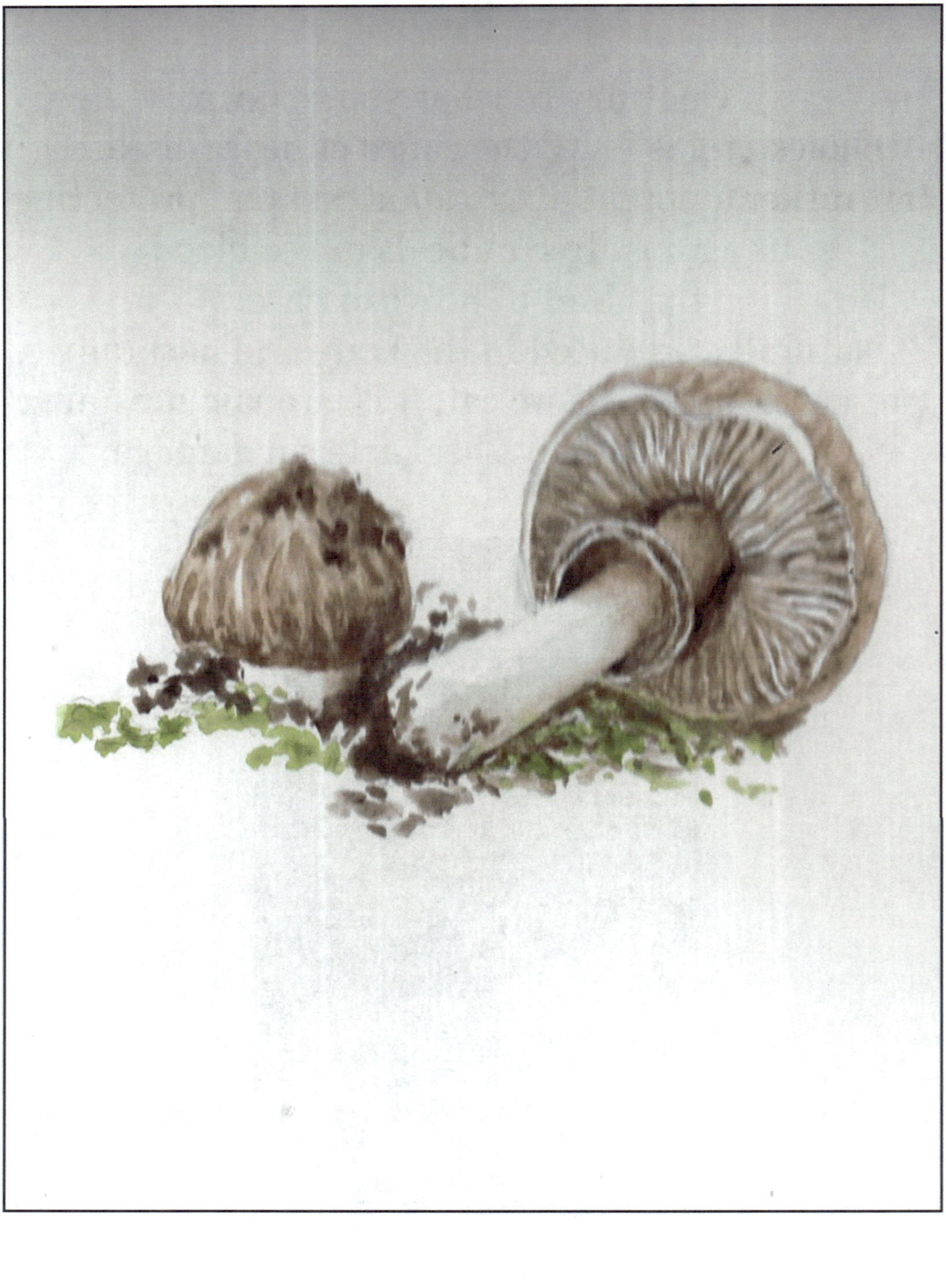

A Shocking Revelation!

I have just received an email that has left me sitting with an open mouth, stunned! One of my colleagues sent it to me just as it was written, by a well-known and respected cardiac surgeon, Dr. Dwight Lundell. I am passing it on, verbatim.

"We physicians with all our training, knowledge and authority often acquire a rather large ego that tends to make it difficult to admit we are wrong. So, here it is. I freely admit to being wrong. As a heart surgeon with twenty-five years' experience, having performed over 5,000 open heart surgeries, today is my day to right the wrong with medical and scientific fact.

"I trained for many years with other prominent physicians labeled "opinion makers." Bombarded with scientific literature, continually attending education seminars, we opinion makers insisted heart disease resulted from the simple fact of elevated blood cholesterol.

The only accepted therapy was prescribing medications to lower cholesterol and a diet that severely restricted fat intake. The latter, of course, we insisted would lower cholesterol and heart disease. Deviations from these recommendations were considered heresy and could quite possibly result in malpractice.

It Is Not Working!

These recommendations are no longer scientifically or morally defensible. The discovery a few years ago that inflammation in the artery wall is the real cause of heart disease is slowly leading to a paradigm shift in how heart disease and other chronic ailments will be treated.

The long-established dietary recommendations have created epidemics of obesity and diabetes, the consequences of which dwarf any historical plague in terms of mortality, human suffering, and dire economic consequences.

Despite the fact that 25% of the population takes expensive statin medications and despite the fact we have reduced the fat content of our diets, more Americans will die this year of heart disease than ever before.

Statistics from the American Heart Association show that 75 million Americans currently suffer from heart disease, 20 million have diabetes, and 57 million are pre-diabetic. These disorders are affecting younger and younger people in greater numbers every year.

Simply stated, without inflammation being present in the body, there is no way that cholesterol would accumulate in the wall of the blood vessel and cause heart disease and strokes. Without inflammation, cholesterol would move freely throughout the body as nature intended. It is inflammation that causes cholesterol to become trapped.

Inflammation is not complicated—it is quite simply your body's natural defense to a foreign invader such as a bacteria, toxin, or virus. The cycle of inflammation is perfect in how it protects your body from these bacterial and viral invaders. However, if we chronically expose the body to injury by toxins or foods the human body was never designed to process, a condition occurs called chronic inflammation. Chronic inflammation is just as harmful as acute inflammation is beneficial.

What thoughtful person would willfully expose himself repeatedly to foods or other substances that are known to cause injury to the body? Well, smokers perhaps, but at least they made that choice willfully.

The rest of us have simply followed the recommended mainstream diet that is low in fat and high in polyunsaturated fats and carbohydrates, not knowing we were causing repeated injury to our blood vessels. This repeated injury created chronic inflammation leading to heart disease, stroke, diabetes, and obesity.

Let me repeat that: The injury and inflammation in our blood vessels is caused by the low-fat diet recommended for years by mainstream medicine.

What are the biggest culprits of chronic inflammation? Quite simply, they are the overload of simple, highly processed carbohydrates (sugar, flour and all the products made from them) and the excess consumption of Omega-6 vegetable oils like soybean, corn, and sunflower that are found in many processed foods.

Take a moment to visualize rubbing a stiff brush repeatedly over soft skin until it becomes quite red and nearly bleeding. You keep this up several times a day, every day for five years. If you could tolerate this painful brushing, you would have a bleeding, swollen infected area that became worse with each repeated injury. This is a good way to visualize the inflammatory process that could be going on in your body right now.

Regardless of wherever the inflammatory process occurs, externally or internally, it is the same. I have peered inside thousands upon thousands of arteries. A diseased artery looks as if someone took a brush and scrubbed repeatedly against its wall. Several times a day, every day, the foods we eat create small injuries compounding into more injuries, causing the body to respond continuously and appropriately with inflammation.

While we savor the tantalizing taste of a sweet roll, our bodies respond alarmingly as if a foreign invader arrived declaring war. Foods loaded with sugars and simple carbohydrates or processed with Omega-6 oils for long shelf life have been the mainstay of the American diet for six decades. These foods have been slowly poisoning everyone.

How does eating a simple sweet roll create a cascade of inflammation to make you sick?

Imagine spilling syrup on your keyboard, and you have a visual of what occurs inside the cell. When we consume simple carbohydrates such as sugar, blood sugar rises rapidly. In response, your pancreas secretes insulin, whose primary purpose is to drive sugar into each cell where it is stored for energy. If the cell is full and does not need glucose, it is rejected to avoid extra sugar gumming up the works.

When your full cells reject the extra glucose, blood sugar rises, producing more insulin, and the glucose converts it to stored fat.

What does all this have to do with inflammation? Blood sugar is controlled in a very narrow range. Extra sugar molecules attach to a variety of proteins that in turn injure the blood vessel wall. This repeated injury to the blood vessel sets off inflammation. When you spike your blood sugar level several times a day, every day, it is exactly like taking sandpaper to the inside of your delicate blood vessels.

While you may not be able to see it, rest assured, it is there. I saw it in over 5,000 surgical patients spanning 25 years who all shared one common denominator—inflammation in their arteries.

Let's get back to the sweet roll. That innocent looking goody not only contains sugars, but it is also baked in one of many Omega-6 oils such as soybean. Chips and fries are soaked in soybean oil; processed foods are manufactured with -6 oils for longer shelf life. While Omega-6s are essential—they are part of every cell membrane controlling what goes in and out of the cell—they must be in the correct balance with Omega-3s. If the balance shifts by consuming excessive Omega-6, the cell membrane produces chemicals called cytokines that directly cause inflammation.

Today's mainstream American diet has produced an extreme imbalance of these two fats. The ratio of imbalance ranges from 15:1 to as high as 30:1 in favor of Omega-6. That's a tremendous amount of cytokines causing inflammation. In today's food environment, a 3:1 ratio would be optimal and healthy.

To make matters worse, the excess weight you are carrying from eating these foods creates overloaded fat cells that pour out large quantities of pro-inflammatory chemicals that add to the injury caused by having high blood sugar. The process that began with a sweet roll turns into a vicious cycle over time that creates heart disease, high blood pressure, diabetes and finally, Alzheimer's disease, as the inflammatory process continues unabated.

There is no escaping the fact that the more we consume prepared and processed foods, the more we trip the inflammation switch little by little each day. The human body cannot process, nor was it designed to consume, foods packed with sugars and soaked in Omega-6 oils.

There is but one answer to quieting inflammation, and that is returning to foods closer to their natural state. To build muscle, eat more protein. Choose carbohydrates that are very complex, such as colorful fruits and vegetables. Cut down on or eliminate inflammation-causing Omega-6 fats such as corn and soybean oil and the processed foods that are made from them.

One tablespoon of corn oil contains 7,280 mg. of Omega-6; soybean contains 6,940 mg. Instead, use olive oil or butter from grass-fed beef.

Animal fats contain less than 20% Omega-6 and are much less likely to cause inflammation than the supposedly healthy oils labelled polyunsaturated. Forget the "science" that has been drummed into your head for decades. The science that saturated fat alone causes heart disease is non-existent. The science that saturated fat raises blood cholesterol is also very weak. Since we now know that cholesterol is not the cause of heart disease, the concern about saturated fat is even more absurd today.

The cholesterol theory led to the no-fat, low-fat recommendations that in turn created the very foods now causing an epidemic of inflammation. Mainstream medicine made a terrible mistake when it advised people to avoid saturated fat in favor of foods high in Omega-6 fats. We now have an epidemic of arterial inflammation leading to heart disease and other silent killers.

What you can do is choose whole foods your grandmother served and not those your mom turned to as grocery store aisles filled with manufactured foods. By eliminating inflammatory foods and adding essential nutrients from fresh unprocessed food, you will reverse years of damage in your arteries and throughout your body from consuming the typical American diet."

The brilliance and courage for a conventional doctor and surgeon to discover, much less admit publicly, that the medical profession has been teaching and practicing in the wrong direction… *has* to be the bravest and most awe-inspiring step he could take! I am so impressed with his ethics and his guts to expose this publicly, that I finished reading it in absolute amazement and appreciation! I am amazed at his fortitude!!! The strength of character and resoluteness that permits one to face opposition unflinchingly; a strong heart in the face of difficulty; the stamina that permits one to expose a long-ingrained belief; the courage that refuses to succumb to an entrenched and consistently marketed misbelief is the most inspiring example of moral integrity that our world desperately needs today!

When a medical doctor veers away from what the medical schools have taught… and he does "natural" healing that opposes standard practice… his license is taken away in order to keep him and others in line, and to keep the public from being aware of other methods…

The Medical Board of the State of Arizona, where he practices, did take his license away. The information is *exactly* what I have been teaching and writing about for the past eight years. The "Naturopathic and Holistic" doctors with whom I have studied gave it to me.

All Our Forbidden Fruits

Just like adults told us when we were children, "Don't eat fish with milk, or you'll get a tummy ache" ... or ..."Step on a crack, you'll break your mother's back" ... or..."Swallow a watermelon seed and it will grow out your ear" ... or ..."Don't open an umbrella in the house or you'll have bad luck" ... or..."Don't let a cat in the room with a new baby or it will suck it's breath"... etc., we have also been given modern dietary myths over and over again, supposedly from knowledgeable authority:

"Don't eat eggs. They are the #1 source of cholesterol! They can lead to heart attacks!"

TRUTH: Dr. Mary Enig (noted world trans-fat authority)

Eggs:

- contain every nutrient the body needs except Vitamin C.
- contain fatty acids, critical to healthy nerve function.
- support brain function.
- contain arachidonic acid, used in cell membranes.
- help counteract inflammation.
- contain lecithin, assisting in assimilation and metabolism of cholesterol.
- contain lutein and zeaxanthin for eye health.
- whites contain the highest quality protein of any food.
- are the second most potent source of vitamin D (yolks).
- Pasture-raised hens produce egg yolks with vitamins A and D... and Omega-3
- DHA (without A and D, you cannot absorb minerals).

TRUTH: Dr. Susan Kleiner

Egg yolks:

- contain acetylcholine, the most abundant neurotransmitter in the body, responsible for every thought and every movement that you have.
- contain phosphatidyl-choline and -serine, which create brain cell channels to allow nutrients in and toxins out.
- Americans eat only 1/3 of their daily need per day, because medical authorities decades ago mistakenly associated eating eggs with elevated blood cholesterol.

TRUTH: Professor Sung I. Koo, Kansas State University, found that a compound in eggs called lecithin reduces the amount of cholesterol your body absorbs.

"Don't eat butter! Margarine is better for you."

TRUTH: The Weston A. Price Foundation

Butter:

- is a rich source of easily absorbed Vitamin A (maintaining good vision).
- also contains all the other fat-soluble vitamins: D, E, and K.
- is rich in important trace minerals: manganese, chromium, zinc, copper, iodine, and selenium (a powerful antioxidant).
- supports immune function, has antimicrobial properties, and aids the intestinal tract.
- provides the perfect balance of Omega-3 fats, which are important for brain function and skin health.
- from grass-fed cows provides Conjugated Linoleic Acid (CLA), a compound that gives excellent protection against cancer and helps build muscle rather than store fat.
- Despite all of the misinformation you may have heard, cholesterol is needed to maintain intestinal health and brain and nervous system development in the young.
- Found only in raw butter, the 'Wulzen Factor' is a hormone-like substance that prevents arthritis and joint stiffness, ensuring that calcium in your body is put into your bones rather than your joints and other tissues. (It is destroyed by pasteurization.)

TRUTH: Dr. Mercola's Internet Newsletter

- Butter contains many nutrients that protect against heart disease: Vitamins A, D, K, and E, lecithin, iodine, and selenium.
- Saturated fats in butter are critical to lung function and protect against asthma.
- Butter helps control weight gain, *yes, weight gain!*
- Vitamin A in butter is essential for proper functioning of the thyroid gland. It is a good source of iodine, helping to prevent goiter in mountainous areas where seafood is not available.
- Many factors in butter ensure optimal growth of children. Low-fat diets in children have been linked to failure to thrive. Yet, low-fat diets are often recommended for youngsters!
- Many nutrients contained in butter are needed for fertility and normal reproduction.

Why you should avoid Margarine, Shortening, and Spreads:

- Trans fats contribute to heart disease, cancer, bone problems, hormonal imbalance, and skin disease; infertility, difficulties in pregnancy, and problems with nursing;
  low birth weight, growth problems, and learning disabilities in children.
- Free radicals and other toxic breakdown products are the result of high temperature industrial processing of vegetable oils.
- Synthetic vitamins are added to margarine.
- The natural color of partially hydrogenated vegetable oil is gray, so manufacturers bleach it to make it white. Yellow coloring is then added to margarine.
- Artificial flavors mask the terrible taste and odor of partially hydrogenated oils.
- Hexane and other toxic solvents are used in the extraction process.

"Only buy pasteurized milk, or you will become ill from harmful bacteria."

TRUTH: Weston A Price Foundation, David Gumpert (*The Raw Milk Revolution*), Dr. Ron Schmid N.D. (*The Untold Story of Milk*), Dr. Francis Pottenger (President American Academy of Applied Nutrition, California),

Randolph Jonnson (Nutrition Consultant, Marin County, California), Dr. Mary Enig

Raw Milk:

- whole milk from grass-fed cows is a complete and balanced food.
- clears children's middle ear infections, and they do not come back.
- clears allergies.
- contains every known fat- and water-soluble vitamin.
- is the chief source of enzymes that facilitate digestion and take work off the pancreas; break down starch, lactose, fat, and phosphate, making milk more digestible, and protect milk from bacterial infection.
- cow's milk has all eight essential amino acids. They are our antibiotic arsenal, providing resistance to many viruses, bacteria, and bacterial toxins.
- is a powerful medicine with naturally occurring hormones and growth factors.
- promotes healthy bone growth and lessens tooth decay.

TRUTH: All these disease fighters are lost when milk is heated to normal pasteurization temperature. Pasteurization destroys or reduces many nutrients in milk, including Vitamins A, C, and B-Complex.

SKIM MILK: By removing important fats and fat-soluble vitamins in the skimming process, skim milk becomes a burden on the body, causing the liver to give up stored nutrients in order to digest it. (The loss of CLA, Vitamin A, and pathogen-busting medium chain triglycerides constitutes an unforgivable crime against nature's perfect food.)

Avoid reduced-fat milk, because manufacturers add powdered eggs and powdered milk (damaged cholesterol products) to skim, 1%, 2%, and low fat milk in order to give them body, but without stating this on the label.

Don't eat salt. It will raise your blood pressure and cause a stroke or heart attack."

TRUTH: Dr. Mary Enig

- *Unrefined* salt is essential to health, activating enzymes needed for brain development and enzymes needed to digest carbohydrate foods: as well as helping your body produce hydrochloric acid for the digestion of meat. Salt also supports adrenal function.

- It's important to pay attention to the kind of salt you use. *Sea salt* contains about 82% sodium chloride, 80 trace minerals, natural iodine and about 14% magnesium, all of which are important to our health.
- Most salt we buy is *highly refined* through an industrial process that uses chemicals and high temperatures to remove valuable magnesium salts and natural trace minerals, while adding several harmful additives, such as aluminum compounds and potassium iodide in amounts that can be toxic to some people. Processors also add a bleaching agent to make it white again. This is the salt we were warned about and have been buying for decades.

"Cholesterol is bad for you. Don't eat fat. It causes heart attacks and strokes."

TRUTH: Dr. Mary Enig

- Contrary to what you've heard, cholesterol is NOT the cause of heart disease, but rather a potent antioxidant weapon protecting us against free radicals in the blood that lead to heart disease. Naturally produced in the body and naturally present in the foods we eat, it is a repair substance that actually helps heal arterial damage.

  High-density lipoproteins (HDL) carry cholesterol away from the cells to the liver, and the low-density lipoproteins (LDL) carry cholesterol to the cells. Both HDL and LDL play critical roles in body chemistry.
- Your body uses cholesterol to manufacture hormones against stress, heart disease, and cancer.
- Your body needs cholesterol to make Vitamin D for bones and the nervous system, muscle tone, insulin, production, reproduction, and the immune system.
- Cholesterol maintains the health of the intestinal wall.
- Mother's milk is especially rich in cholesterol to ensure proper development of the brain and nervous system.
- It is needed for proper function of serotonin receptors ("feel good") in the brain.
- Cholesterol also helps the repair of damaged cells.

However, heat and oxygen can damage cholesterol by damaging fats. These are the trans fats and hydrogenated fats that are so destructive to our bodies.

TRUTH: Dr. Russell Blaylock (Neurosurgeon)

- Cholesterol is NOT the cause of arteriosclerosis.
- The number one cause is over-consumption of dietary Omega-6 fatty acids such as canola, soybean, corn, safflower, sunflower, and cottonseed oil.
- These are hydrogenated fats and oils that become oxidized and create Lp(a), a lipoprotein which clings to the inner veins as plaque.

Please don't believe everything you read. Most of the misinformation we receive is for the monetary gain of one corporation or another. Do intelligent research. Your family's life and health depend upon it.

Amazing Bee Pollen

A "miracle food" from the beehive, bee pollen, is an effective natural preventative: a POWERHOUSE! It contains all the vitamins, minerals, amino acids (proteins), enzymes, carbohydrates, hormones, essential fatty acids, and trace minerals known to be needed for our human nutrition.

It cannot be synthesized in a laboratory. Only the bee can pollinate plants to extract the mysterious extra factor that gives bee pollen its incredible nutritional factors. Also, bee pollen contains a live electric charge. When worker bees leave the hive, they have a slightly negative or neutral charge. When returning to the hive, the same bees register a positive charge of electricity as much as 1.5 volts. The live energized bee pollen they carry is also electrically charged.

Pollen is the live male spore of all botanicals and is necessary for fertilization and growth of the species. We could not live without bees to pollinate our plants and give us plant food... and animals could not live without that food either… so we would not have animal protein, and thus, without food, life would come to an end. Yet, our commercial agriculture proponents spray with pesticides and herbicides and the toxins that are killing bees and demolishing bee hives! What a crime!

Want a shock? Adult worker bees subsist on honey and live a few weeks, but the Queen Bee lives five or six years! What does she eat? An exclusive diet of Royal jelly (produced from bee pollen). She becomes far superior to the workers of the hive. Bee pollen contains a rejuvenating, health-promoting, and life-extending force. The tiny larvae are fed bee pollen to ensure a good start in life, but one of the single larvae (identical in every way to its sister larvae) is transformed by Royal jelly into the royalty of the hive… the Queen Bee.

Professor Dr. Nikolai V. Tsitsin, a Russian botanist and biologist, investigated the lifestyle of centenarians past 125 years of age living in the Caucasus Mountains of upper Russia. Many were beekeepers and ate the sticky residue (bee pollen) found on the bottom of the hives as a principal food. Tsitsin was impressed with the *quality* of their lives, too. All of these people were actively working and in good health in spite of their advanced age!

Another Russian scientist, Dr. Naum P. Yoirich, stated, "Bee pollen is one of the original treasure-houses of nutrition and medicine. Long lives are attained by bee pollen users. It contains every important substance necessary to life."

Scientists at the Far East Institute of the Soviet Union in Vladivostok concluded, "Bee pollen has regenerative properties for the body. Bee pollen contains all the amino acids, mineral salts, vitamins, and enzymes in perfect proportion as needed by the organism."

Dr. Alain Callais, Paris, stated that bee pollen is richer in essential protein than any animal source and said it contains more amino acids than meat, eggs, or cheese of equal weight. Yugoslav researchers at the University of Sarajevo used oral bee pollen therapy on a group of impotent men. After a thirty-day period, over half were documented with an increase in production of sperm. Bee pollen's gonadotropic hormones act as a reproductive gland stimulant.

A German/Swiss team of urologists reported bee pollen ingestion proved most successful as a treatment of prostatitis and prevented the need for surgery.

In 1948, the *Journal of the National Cancer Institute* published results that determined bee pollen contains an active anticancer element with the power to slow the development of mammary tumors, concluding it is a powerful cancer fighter that can be added to food. The University of Vienna reported a *noticeable decrease in the side effects of radiation therapy* on women with uterine cancer, when bee pollen was added to their diet. Hair loss, nausea and vomiting, loss of appetite, and bladder and rectal inflammations were greatly reduced in the women who took bee pollen during the course of their radiation therapy.

In his popular book, *About Pollen*, author Carlson Wade says, "The healing, rejuvenating, and disease-fighting effects of this total nutrient are hard to believe, yet are fully documented. Aging, digestive upsets, prostate disease, sore throats, acne, fatigue, sexual problems, allergies, and a host of other problems have been successfully treated using bee pollen."

It is important you always buy raw, unheated pollen. It is important you know and can trust the source of your bee pollen. A good source is from clean, sun-washed, high mountains and deserts of the West, and many good bee pollens are available blended from different regions of the Midwest. Avoid those imported from Spain or China, some of which are heat-treated, and also because of their questionable sources.

Russian research shows Royal jelly contains *acetylcholine*, an important element shown to be lacking in the brains of Alzheimer's disease victims. Royal jelly regulates blood pressure, stimulates suprarenal glands, and enhances the immune system. It is effective in cases of arteriosclerosis and coronary deficiency, reduces cholesterol, and restores energy where it is lacking.

I do not know what you have gathered from all of this, but to me, if the Queen Bee lives five or six years on Royal jelly, and the worker bees live several weeks on honey, it caused me to run right to my health food store and buy Royal jelly. I always use myself as a guinea pig first, when finding a new breakthrough… and I sure am enjoying a teaspoon every day… yum, yum.

Build Immunity for Freedom from Disease

It is wintertime again, and everyone is worrying about getting the flu, or a bad cold with a sore throat and coughing. Flu shots are advertised in every media, and signs are in the front windows of pharmacies. It is sad that we accept that precept to keep our bodies free from illness, since it has not been too successful and has had side effects. You can avoid illness this season with knowledge of food, vitamins, and minerals that will keep you well, instead of imbibing harmful pharmaceutical drugs.

Vitamin C is *the* immunity-building front runner! A MINIMUM of 3000 milligrams of Vitamin C (ascorbic acid) spaced throughout the day is a necessity. I hear from my readers and students that they take Vitamin C in their multivitamins, but if you look at the amount on your bottle, you will find it is not enough. There is no limit to the amount you can safely take. Dr. Linus Pauling, who in 1970 discovered his "Unified Vitamin C Theory," died in 2013 at the age of 94 and was taking 18,000 mg. a day.

Vitamin C stimulates the production of Collagen, which is the most abundant protein built in our bodies, laced through our ligaments, cartilage, and connective tissues… building healthy bones and firmness of skin. Vitamin C promotes infection-fighting white blood cells; builds vein and capillary strength; aids brain and heart health; is a key factor in treating diabetes, high blood pressure, and male infertility; decreases risk of gout and gallstones; is an aid to asthma and allergies; prevents and reduces shingles; helps flush out toxins, heavy metals such as lead and mercury, pesticides, and petrochemicals; safeguards against radiation poisoning; greatly reduces the risk of developing cancer… intravenous large doses treat or slow down cancer.

Dr. Jonathan Wright of the Tacoma Clinic in Washington says intravenous doses heal chicken pox and measles, which no drug can cure. Vitamin E and green tea work together with Vitamin C and boost antioxidant activity. Vitamin C is depleted by tobacco, Aspirin, oral contraceptives, and the antibiotic, Tetracycline.

Foods: Citrus fruits, green and red bell peppers, tomatoes, celery, dark greens, broccoli, cauliflower, papaya, strawberries, pineapple, persimmons, and potatoes. For years, the medical profession has warned us not to consume oils and fats, so we have been plagued with illnesses commensurate with a low-fat diet. The truth is that Essential Fatty Acids are *essential* for our bodies' health… our bodies can't make them. We must eat fats and oils for our bodies' function.

But it must be healthy fats and oils, not the detrimental ones. Organic coconut oil, olive oil, walnut oil, macadamia oil, and butter are natural, healthy oils and are necessary for the absorption of the fat-soluble vitamins A, D, E, and K.

Fat is the most abundant substance in our body, next to water. More than 70% of brain and nerve cells are fat. Every cell membrane is 30% fat. Fat is essential for growth in babies and children. Fat provides energy to the heart. Saturated fat protects the liver from toxins such as alcohol and Tylenol. Lungs cannot work effectively without saturated fats. Saturated fat is needed for calcium to make bone.

Partially hydrogenated and hydrogenated oils: corn, soybean, canola, safflower, sunflower, and cottonseed oils are detrimental Omega-6… are chemically altered, and the first three are genetically modified (GMO's), and they are in almost every processed food in grocery stores. Please read the ingredients on the *back* of the bag, can, or box before purchasing it. It takes nine months to rid the body of these fats.

Animal fat from *wild* animals and *grass-fed* animals is healthy fat; not the fat from animals in feed lots for the last eight months of their lives. Only fat from poultry that is pasture-raised is healthy, not from those in contained barns. Fish that is caught wild, preferably in Alaska or the North Pacific, is healthy; while farm-raised fish are not. The meat, bones, skin, and fat from these animals are all requisites for true health. Eating skinless, boneless does not cut it.

Omega-3 fatty acids are also a huge deterrent to disease, containing DHA for brain functioning and EPA for heart, cell, and joint functioning. Omega-3 reduces inflammation, which is the primary cause of all diseases. It calms inflammation of Crohn's disease and ulcerative colitis, improves blood vessel function, lowers blood pressure, decreases risk of cardiovascular disease, prevents blood clots, helps prevent atrial fibrillation, reduces, depression, is beneficial for eczema, along with kidneys and lungs, and it aids fertility in men and women, wound healing, cognitive function and clear memory.

It is important during pregnancy for a baby's neurological, mental, and emotional health, and future learning ability. (It has been suggested that a mother's lack of Omega-3 may be one of the causes of autism and ADHD in a child.)

Sources of Omega-3 are anchovies, sardines, salmon, walnuts, purslane, pumpkin seeds, brassicas such as broccoli and cauliflower, kale, spinach, flaxseed, hemp, and chia seeds.

Omega-3 supplements are needed along with food that supplies them. Krill oil is the best to purchase, as it is found in the waters of the Antarctic, is the smallest crustacean in the ocean, and doesn't contain mercury.

I choose to buy raw milk rather than pasteurized milk. Pasteurized milk is boiled twice, and most of the nutritional elements are boiled out. Raw milk is a complete and balanced food. It provides every water- and fat-soluble vitamin, mineral, enzyme, and amino acid. Raw milk clears allergies, and children's middle ear infections disappear and do not re-appear. It is a valuable healing food, a powerful medicine with naturally occurring hormones and growth factors. You could literally live on raw milk alone for your entire life.

Most people are not bothered by raw milk like they are with pasteurized milk, because the lactase in raw milk counteracts the lactose that upsets some stomachs, and the casein in milk is counteracted by a protein in raw milk. Look online for Dr. Weston A. Price to learn more about raw milk and enter your zip code to find a dairy near you that sells it.

Bone broth is one of the most nutritional foods for immunity. I buy organic chicken and simmer it for twenty-four hours. Add a few eggshells into your broth while simmering, because the membrane in the shell builds synovial fluid that keeps your joints moving easily. Also add chicken feet to supply you with extra cartilage.

I buy pasture-fed beef bones for beef broth, and simmer seventy-two hours, adding a bit of hot water when it seems to evaporate. Add ½ cup of apple cider vinegar to every gallon of water. During the last hour, I add celery, carrots, parsley, and onions for flavor. When done, I put the pot in the fridge and save the congealed fat to cook with, storing it in the freezer. I pour the broth through a strainer or sieve into jars, freezing them for the future. (This way, no pieces of bones are in the broth.) This broth can be the base of soups or stews instead of store-bought, which does not have the same value and also contains harmful preservatives and additives. I keep a jar in my fridge to take a tablespoon or two for nourishment.

Vitamin D3 has come into the limelight as essential for more than just building bone. The broad spectrum of diseases affected by Vitamin

D3 intake is staggering. It is a critical fat-soluble vitamin and works with Vitamin A to utilize calcium and phosphorus in building bones and teeth. Twenty minutes outside in the sun in the morning provides you with the amount your need, preferable between 10 A.M. and 3 P.M… but without that, you need a supplement of 5000IU to meet the necessary levels. If you are getting Vitamin D3 from a supplement, take Vitamin K with it.

Dr. Jonathan Wright of the Tacoma Clinic in Washington calls this the "Diabetes Vitamin," lowering the risk of Diabetes Type 2. He adds that it reduces the risk of fractures and falls by improving muscle and bone strength, controls blood pressure, drives depression away, prevents flu and pneumonia, stimulates the genes that starve cancer cells, and helps stop the spread of those cancer cells.

Dr. Andrew Weil said it prevents Diabetes Type 1, is vital to proper immune function and disease prevention, builds bones… reducing osteoporosis and hip fracture, reduces cancers by 50%, and prevents auto-immune disorders, particularly multiple sclerosis, and rheumatoid arthritis.

Vitamin D3 is an important factor in mental cognition, cutting the risk for Alzheimer's and Parkinson's, helping relieve headaches, aiding sleep, lifting mood, and helping heal depression (including SAD I areas with a lot of rain and lack of sun).

Dr. Matthias Rath says it is essential for optimal calcium metabolism in artery walls, including removal of calcium from atherosclerotic deposits. Vitamin D3 strengthens the heart and reduces risk of stroke.

Sunscreen with 15 SPF reduces Vitamin D3 by 95%. Fifteen to twenty minutes of sun does not cause Melanoma. It takes a lot longer to cause sunburn. Vitamin B Complex, Vitamin E, and minerals: Potassium, Zinc, Magnesium and Selenium, Amino Acids and Enzymes are all important elements, too. Do some studying to promote a joyous life.

Energy and good health are worth a fortune.

Eggs, The Differences You Need to Know

This nutritious, delicious food has been maligned for years, partly because of ignorance, and partly because of dishonesty that is in bed with greed. Eggs have been portrayed as "bad for our cholesterol," one more nail in the coffin to frighten the public into buying statins to lower our cholesterol count.

Dr. Susan Kleiner says, "Americans eat one-third of their daily needs per day because medical authorities mistakenly associated eating eggs with elevated cholesterol, decades ago. To the contrary, eggs contain lecithin, assisting in the proper assimilation and metabolism of cholesterol and other fat constituents and, also, trace minerals."

So states Dr. Mary Enig, the prime authority on trans-fats which have been a major cause of degenerative diseases in today's world. "Eggbeaters," advertised as the solution to eating eggs and not getting sick, are *really* a fabricated product that are made with the very vegetable oil against which Dr. Enig warns us.

In truth, eggs support brain function, help build prostaglandin to counteract inflammation, and contain lutein and zeaxanthin for eye health. The choline in eggs is critical to healthy nerve function, clearing fatty liver and aiding HDL, LDL, and triglycerides. They also contain arachidonic acid, a fat used in cell membranes.

Dr. Susan Kleiner says, "The acetylcholine in eggs is the most abundant neurotransmitter in the body, responsible for every thought and every movement that we have. Phosphatidyl-choline in the egg yolks create brain cell channels to allow nutrients in and toxins out."

Those are certainly compelling reasons to eat eggs.

It is important to buy eggs from pasture-fed chickens. These chickens are out in the healing sun, scratching in the dirt and stones, and eating grains, grass, worms, and other insects. The best way to get these eggs is to buy them from a farmer or a farmer's market. Very few towns, large or small, do not have farmers' markets. Eggs purchased from grocery stores are usually from giant factory chicken farms, where standard industry practice is to wash eggs. Washed eggs spoil faster, so they coat eggs with oil. It is akin to adding preservatives to processed foods.

What is on the outside of the shell is as important as what is inside. Eggshells are a porous membrane like our skin with approximately 7,500 pores per egg. What goes on the shell can end up in your egg.

The big producers raise thousands of chickens in one huge barn, and then say on the carton that these eggs are cage-free or free roaming. They are sprayed with antibiotics to keep disease down, and are fed the wrong feed, sometimes containing animal by-products. Most of the "free-range" chickens only have "access" to the outdoors; their free-range criteria provide tiny, enclosed porches with roofs and concrete or wood flooring. There is no way that thousands of chickens are going to fit in that small cubicle. And, since the chickens were hatched in the barn, and their feed and water are inside, it is rare for them to want to go elsewhere. Only 5% of hens are allowed to roam "cage free." What you want to look for is: pasture fed and 100% organic. 100% organic eggs are fed a hormone-free diet.

Dr. Mercola advised us by email recently that Tyson injects chickens, before hatching, with antibiotics and labels them "raised without antibiotics."

There is no nutritional difference between brown and white eggs: however, Omega-3 is only found in the yolks. Other than using egg whites in meringue for pies, you should always eat the whole egg. The advertising you have seen that tells you to make scrambled eggs from only egg whites is nutritionally erroneous.

Pasture fed eggs contain: 1/4 less saturated fat, 2/3 more Vitamin A, 2 times more Omega-3 fatty acids (ALA and DHA), 3 times more Vitamin E, 7 times more beta carotene, and 1/3 less cholesterol.

We have been led to believe that raw eggs are dangerous harbingers of salmonella poisoning. That can be another piece of misinformation. Dr. Mercola has two raw eggs in his morning smoothie every day. I mix my homemade mayonnaise with only a pasture-fed raw egg, since I'm uneasy about eggs purchased at the grocery store that I'm not going to cook. Cal-Maine, Inc., the largest egg distributors/packers in the United States, recalled 288,000 eggs in November 2010 due to salmonella.

In fact, the British found that 23% of farms with caged hens tested positive for salmonella, compared to just over 4% in organic flocks and 6.5% in pasture-raised flocks.

You can still depend on your small, local farmer to produce some of the best food on earth. I buy mine from two FFA boys at 4:00 PM each Tuesday in front of our library. The egg yolks are deeper yellow than the grocery store variety, and they taste so much better.

To locate a free-range pasture farm near you, try:

- www.eatwild.com
- www.localharvest.org

Enjoy the Health Benefits of Coconut Oil

Coconut oil is the purest oil available. It enters the body as energy, instead of turning into stored fat. Coconut oil also improves your immune system. It is important that it is untreated virgin organic coconut oil.

Don't you wonder, as I do, why this information is being kept quiet? Who gains from our pain? Who sweeps it under the carpet?

HAIR CARE: Coconut oil helps healthy hair growth, providing natural shine, and is effective in reducing protein loss in damaged hair. Coconut oil is extensively used in the Indian sub-continent. Most of the people in these countries apply coconut oil to their hair daily after a bath.

It is an excellent conditioner and helps in the regrowth of damaged hair. Regular head massage with coconut oil ensures your scalp is free of dandruff, even if your scalp is dry. It is used in manufacturing various conditioners and dandruff relief creams.

SKIN CARE: Coconut oil is an excellent skin massage cream. It acts as an effective moisturizer on all types of skin, including dry skin. After bathing, apply it to your whole body and then dry with a towel. It makes your skin moist without causing it to be oily. It delays wrinkles, sagging of skin, and helps prevent aging. It is also a suntan lotion without the harmful chemicals that block the pores, causing the prevalent skin cancer we see now.

Coconut oil also helps in treating various skin problems, including psoriasis, dermatitis, eczema, and other skin infections. Therefore, coconut oil forms the basic ingredient of various body care products such as soaps, lotions, creams, etc., used for skin care.

HEART DISEASES: There has been a gross misconception that coconut oil is bad for the heart, because it contains a large quantity of saturated fats. This misconception has aided producers of harmful vegetable oil to move coconut oil off the market for forty years.

Dr. Mary Enig, the world's trans-fat authority, says, "Saturated fats protect body organs."

Coconut oil contains 50% lauric acid, which helps to prevent various heart problems, including high cholesterol levels and high blood pressure. Coconut oil does not increase LDL, sticky lipoprotein, like Omega-6 vegetable oils, which are the primary cause of plaque in the arteries.

Saturated fats provide energy to the heart in times of stress. Studies have shown that saturated fats are the heart's preferred food, which is why a concentration of saturated fat is in the tissues surrounding the heart. It also reduces the incidence of injury in arteries and therefore helps to prevent atherosclerosis.

DIGESTION: Internal use of coconut oil occurs primarily as cooking and baking oil. Coconut oil helps in improving the digestive system, and thus prevents various stomach and digestion-related problems, including irritable bowel syndrome. The saturated fats present in coconut oil have antimicrobial properties and help in dealing with various bacteria, fungi, parasites, etc., that cause indigestion. It also helps in absorption of other nutrients such as vitamins, minerals, and amino acids.

IMMUNITY: The main medium-chain fatty acid in coconut oil is lauric acid, a proven antiviral, antibacterial, and antifungal agent that is also found in mother's milk. Converted in your body to a substance called monolaurin, it helps you defend against viruses, bacteria, and other pathogens, and strengthens your immune system, protecting you from a wide range of diseases.

Highly protective lauric acid should be called a "conditionally essential fatty acid" because it is made only by the mammary gland and not in the liver like other saturated fats. It comes from just three dietary sources: in small amounts, butterfat – in large amounts, coconut oil and palm kernel oil. Coconut oil also helps in preventing degenerative diseases due to its antioxidant properties.

HEALING AND INFECTIONS: When applied to infections, it forms a chemical layer which protects the infected body part from external dust, air, fungi, bacteria, and virus. Coconut oil is most effective on bruises, as it speeds up the healing process by repairing damaged tissues. When antibiotics are losing ground to infectious organisms, nature has provided an antibiotic to which germs cannot develop a resistance.

The lauric acid in coconut oil is known to fight:

- Viruses: HIV, measles, herpes, mononucleosis, hepatitis C, and AIDS.
- Bacteria: pneumonia, earache, food poisoning, meningitis, stomach ulcers, rheumatic fever, gonorrhea.
- Parasites: intestinal infections.
- Fungi and yeast: ringworm, candida, athlete's foot, diaper rash, and thrush.

LIVER: Saturated fats protect the liver from toxins such as alcohol and Tylenol and prevent the accumulation of fat. Today, as people shun saturated fats like coconut oil and eat more polyunsaturated oils, liver problems have become more common.

BRAIN: 60% of your brain is composed of fat. Phospholipids contain 50% saturated fat and make up the brain cell membranes. They generally contain one saturated fat and one unsaturated fat. You nourish your brain cells when you eat saturated fats, and when you don't eat enough saturated fats, the chemistry of the brain may be compromised.

KIDNEY: Coconut oil helps to prevent kidney and gall bladder diseases. It also helps to dissolve kidney stones. Omega-3 fatty acids, saturated fats, and cholesterol all work together synergistically to maintain normal kidney function, which is critical for managing blood pressure and filtering toxins from the body.

Coconut oil also enhances kidney function by providing a saturated fatty acid called myristic acid, which plays a vital role in the biochemistry of the kidneys. In a key reaction called "myristolation," myristic acid is added to a protein. This process allows the cells of the kidney to communicate with each other.

LUNGS: The lungs cannot work without adequate saturated fats in the diet. This is because the fatty acids in the lung surfactant (a fluid that enables the lungs to work) are normally 100% saturated. When people consume a lot of partially hydrogenated fats and vegetable oils, trans-fatty acids, and polyunsaturated fatty acids, the lungs cannot work effectively.

These damaged Omega-6 oils contribute to the rising incidence of asthma in children, while children who consume ample amounts of butterfat and coconut oil have much lower rates of asthma. In fact, changes in fat consumption patterns over the past forty years explain the rising incidence of all types of lung disease, including asthma and lung cancer.

BONES: Coconut oil improves the ability of our bodies to absorb important minerals, including calcium and magnesium, which are necessary for the development of bones. Thus, coconut oil is very useful to women who are prone to osteoporosis after middle age.

DENTAL CARE: Calcium is an important element present in teeth. Since coconut oil facilitates absorption of calcium by the body, it aids in building strong teeth. Coconut oil also stops tooth decay. A new practice has been found to stop plaque on teeth. First thing in the morning, before drinking water or brushing teeth, squish coconut oil through the teeth for 15-45 minutes before spitting it out.

ALZHEIMER'S DISEASE: Dr. Mary Newport healed her husband's Alzheimer's in several months' time by giving him four tablespoons of coconut oil in his morning oatmeal each day. The only time he lapsed was if he accidentally skipped a day, and she had to start it all over again.

Coconut oil disappeared from the grocery shelves in the 1970's because the American Soybean Association wanted to make more profit and took out a multi-million-dollar advertising campaign knocking coconut oil; and the American public believed them, as we have with most misleading marketing since that time. And harmful hydrogenated trans-fats made their appearance and altered our health and immunity.

Make coconut oil a main staple in your diet and reclaim your barrier to disease.

The Fundamental Amino Acids

Amino acids are absolutely necessary for life, growth, and healing. The body uses them to break down food and repair tissue. They create the acid/alkaline balance of tissues and blood. Our liver produces 80% of our amino acids, our food produces 20%.

The twenty-nine amino acids are known building blocks of protein in the body. Animal protein is the only source of *complete* amino acids. Sources of proteins from the vegetable kingdom like legumes, beans, nuts, cereals, and grains contain only incomplete protein; that is, they are low in one or more essential amino acids. They should be eaten together and combined with at least a small amount of animal protein.

Most grain-based cuisines instinctively incorporate this principle. For example, animal products plus corn and beans are staple fare in Mexican cuisine, as are chickpeas and whole wheat in the Middle East.

Protein cannot be adequately utilized without dietary fats. That is why protein and fats occur together in eggs, milk, fish, and meats. A high protein and low-fat diet can cause many problems, including depletion of Vitamin A and D reserves.

Vegetarians often claim that animal products shorten life span, but a look at peoples who have the longest life span: Russians from the Caucasus Mountains, Soviet Georgian populations, Vilcabamba people in Peru, and Pakistani Hunzas all show that those who have the most meat and fat in their diets live the longest.

The vegetarian inhabitants of southern India have one of the shortest life spans in the world.

Our bodies cannot produce the nine *essential* aminos. They must come from the nutrients we consume. (Bee pollen contains all the essential aminos.) Here are the essential aminos and the food sources and benefits of each:

Histidine: Rice, wheat, rye. Promotes tissue growth and repair, protects against radiation damage, lowers blood pressure, stimulates stomach acid, and may improve sexual function.

Isoleucine: Almonds, cashews, chicken, chickpeas, eggs, fish, lentils, liver, meat, rye, most seeds. Required for hemoglobin formation, stabilizes and regulates blood sugar and energy levels, enhances endurance, repairs muscle tissue.

Leucine: Brown rice, beans, meat, nuts, whole wheat. Source of fuel, promotes healing of bones, skin, and muscle tissue, increases growth hormone production, lowers elevated blood sugar levels.

Lysine: Cheese, eggs, fish, lima beans, milk, potatoes, red meat, yeast. Fights cold sores and herpes viruses, promotes calcium absorption, bone development and growth in children, collagen formation, and tissue repair.

Methionine: Beans, eggs, fish, garlic, lentils, meat, onions, seeds, yogurt. Helps prevent fat buildup in liver and arteries, aids in digestion, removes heavy metal toxins, fights muscle weakness, prevents brittle hair, protects against radiation damage.

Phenylalanine: Beef, poultry, pork, fish, milk, yogurt, eggs, cheese. Promotes action of central nervous system, may elevate mood and decrease pain, aids in memory and learning, helps suppress appetite.

Threonine: Dairy, eggs, meat, wheat germ, nuts, beans, seeds, some vegetables. Helps maintain body's protein balance, aids liver function, enhances immune system, aids in formation of collagen, elastin, and tooth enamel.

Tryptophan: Brown rice, cottage cheese, meat, peanuts. Needed for production of niacin and serotonin, combats depression and insomnia, helps stabilize mood, aids in weight control.

Valine: Dairy, grains, meat, mushrooms, peanuts. Used in muscle metabolism, tissue repair, and nitrogen balance.

Amino acids are to be taken on an empty stomach, at least a half hour before eating. Food competes and reduces their absorption.

Poor diet, unhealthy habits, and environmental pollutants mean that the "essential amino acids" our body cannot produce may not be sufficient to produce the "non-essentials." This can be corrected by increasing intake of protein foods or supplements.

Amino acids work well with other natural healers: herbs, minerals, and antioxidants.

Green Superfoods

Superfoods are superior sources of essential nutrients we need but cannot make ourselves. Our mineral-depleted soils since the 1950's make Chlorella and Spirulina nutritionally more potent than regular foods. These green and blue-green algae superfoods have rich, high-quality protein, fiber, chlorophyll, vitamins, minerals, enzymes, and all the essential amino acids our bodies can't manufacture. They are the richest plant sources of Vitamin B12. They are the only food source (other than mother's milk) of GLA, an essential fatty acid. They are the most potent source of beta carotene available in the world today. They stimulate immune response, accelerate healing and tissue repair, help prevent degenerative disease, and promote longer life.

Chlorella is a single-cell algae from lake water. Chlorella alone has a higher concentration of chlorophyll than any known plant. All its natural properties function together in a way that individual supplements cannot touch. It is a complete protein food, with Vitamins A, B1, B2, B6, C, E, magnesium, zinc, calcium, iron, potassium, lipoic acid, and many minerals high enough to be considered supplemental amounts. It is called "Nature's Multivitamin."

Cholrella:

- it's cell wall material is especially beneficial for intestinal and bowel health, detoxifying the colon, stimulating peristaltic activity, and promoting friendly bacteria.
- eliminates heavy metals, such as lead, mercury, copper, and cadmium.
- binds to harmful pesticides and insecticides such as PCB's and DDT, involved in breast cancer and carries them out of the body.
- strengthens the liver, your body's major detoxifying organ, to rid you of infective agents.
- chlorophyll improves immunity, alkalinity, and inflammation.
- reduces pain associated with fibromyalgia.
- normalizes blood pressure.
- helps lower over-all body fat.
- reduces arthritis stiffness.
- helps reduce fatigue from viral infections such as Epstein-Barr and herpes.
- relieves indigestion, hiatal hernia, gastritis, and ulcers.
- decreases menopausal complaints by assisting with estrogen production in the body.

- is effective in weight loss programs. Its rich nutrition keeps energy up during dieting and maintains muscle during periods of lower food intake.
- is a key addition to your anti-cancer arsenal.

Spirulina is a microscopic green alga harvested in both ocean and lake waters. It can be cultivated in extreme environments useless for conventional agriculture. Small-scale community farms are spirulina's biggest producers. It grows in such a variety of climates and conditions that some consider it the nutritional answer for whole populations on the brink of starvation.

It does not deplete any topsoil and doubles its biomass every two to five days. Researchers say that spirulina alone could double the protein available to people on a fraction of the world's land, while helping restore the environmental balance of the planet.

Spirulina:

- yields twenty times more protein than soybeans, forty times more protein than corn, and 400 times more protein than beef, accelerating healing.
- is a complete protein with all twenty-two amino acids, the entire Vitamin B-complex, including B12 (with more than liver), carotenes, naturally chelated minerals, and essential fatty acids such as gamma linolenic acid (GLA).
- affords high digestibility for both rapid and long-range energy.
- is an especially rich source of iron (twenty-eight times higher than beef liver) to help rebuild red blood cells. Spirulina reduces your risk of cancer, especially mouth cancer.
- can also be used as a rich source of nutrients to help the body heal and overcome the damaging effects of chemotherapy.
- demonstrates amazing activity against AIDS.
- is a good choice for weight loss.
- helps lower cholesterol.
- aids stamina strength.
- boosts infection-fighting production for immune protection.
-

Please think about adding these two Superfoods to your regimen, like I have, and multiply your health benefits many times over. To me, these tiny pills are absolutely amazing!

Healing Vegetables, Fruits, Nuts, and Seeds

We are told to eat our fruits and vegetables. To gain nutrition from them, they need to be devoid of pesticides. Those that are the lowest in sprayed pesticides are: onions, pineapples, avocados, asparagus, sweet peas, mangoes, eggplant, cantaloupe (domestic), kiwi, cabbage, watermelon, sweet potatoes, grapefruit, and mushrooms. Corn is low also, but since 95% of corn is genetically modified, it is a 'no-no' and out of the running.

"The Dirty Dozen" are the highest in pesticides, and it is a good idea to use your 'organic' dollars here: apples and pears, celery, strawberries, peaches, spinach, nectarines, grapes (imported), sweet bell peppers, potatoes, blueberries, lettuce, kale, and collard greens.

Berries that are from South America may be raised organically, but when their ships land in our ports, we open up the holds and spray them with pesticides as a rule. If the berries come from Mexico, it is safer, because they do not come by ship, but by truck and train.

Your best bet, health-wise, is to buy organic produce as a regular habit, and the best and easiest way to do this is to buy both produce and meats at your farmer's markets. It is rare to find a farmer who uses chemical pesticides and insecticides there. The labels may not say 'organic', but they farm organically. It is so expensive and time consuming to follow our government regulations to get the "organic certification," that they raise edibles safely but do not spend the time or money to comply for the certificate.

It probably will surprise you to know that celery is one of the highest in all-around nutrients, followed by spinach and kale. It includes protein, fiber, calcium, iron, magnesium, phosphorus, potassium, sodium, zinc, vitamins A, B6, C, E, and K, thiamine, riboflavin, niacin, and folate. Now, doesn't that surprise you? Who would guess that those quiet everyday greens could hold so much nutrition?

Here are some quick fixes from your garden:

- Aching joints: tart cherries.
- Age spots: 1/4 cup yogurt plus one teaspoon horseradish.
- Allergies: cranberries.
- Arthritis: macadamias and walnuts.
- Asthma: grapefruit (but, if you are taking pharmaceutical drugs, you

had better check with your doctor, because grapefruit doubles the efficacy of the drugs).

- Burns: aloe, a cut onion, flour (just put your hand or burnt part into the flour before you do anything else).
- Candida: coconut oil (eats fungus).
- Cholesterol: dark chocolate, avocados.
- Constipation: dandelions.
- Cuts: honey.
- Dark under-eye circles: one tablespoon turmeric plus one tablespoon honey (10 minutes).
- Depression: salmon.
- Diabetes: cinnamon, green coffee beans.
- Diarrhea: peeled apple.
- Digestion: artichokes, papaya, or pineapple before a meal.
- Even skin tone: rub on carrot juice.
- Estrogen breakdown: cauliflower.
- Folate: lentils.
- Good bowels: an apple a day.
- Gout: black cherry juice.
- High blood pressure: bok choy, celery (it is said that eight stalks of celery a day will lower your blood pressure to normal in one year's time).
- Hot flashes: vanilla pudding.
- Inflammation: fennel seeds, ginger, turmeric, cayenne pepper.
- Memory: beans, eggs, blueberries.
- Night vision: squash.
- Prostate: Brazil nuts.
- Risk of stroke: apricots (not dried with sulfur).
- Tiredness: beans, celery, cucumber, organic meat, raw milk.
- Vision: mango, corn, egg yolks, butterfat.
- Weak bones: Brussels sprouts.
-

There are many more foods that heal... but only if they are organic, real foods, and not processed in bottles, jars, boxes, bags, or cans. When food processing companies have altered them to be sold in grocery stores, they have been compromised with additives, preservatives, coloring, synthetics, GMO's, MSG, high fructose corn syrup, hydrogenated trans-fats, Equal, Splenda, sugars, and salts (not sea salt); and this is done for the manufacturers benefit...

to give the product a long shelf life... (and to our detrimen: illness).

Here are some of the benefits of eating fresh produce:

- Aids digestion: artichokes, chili peppers, flax, mangoes, pineapple, peaches.
- Protects heart: apples, bananas, cherries, blueberries, carrots, chestnuts, beets, broccoli, artichokes, cabbage, olive oil, rice, lemons, limes, oranges, green tea, flax, grapes, prunes, tomatoes, walnuts.
- Improves lung capacity: apples.
- Boosts memory: blueberries, figs, walnuts, prunes, strawberries.
- Blocks diarrhea: bananas, pineapple.
- Combats cancer: apricots, blueberries, cabbage, broccoli, cherries, figs, carrots, chili peppers, cantaloupe, beans, lemons, limes, green tea, oats, rice, onions, garlic, oranges, peaches, tomatoes, walnuts, grapes, olive oil, sweet potatoes, chestnuts, mushrooms. (Grapefruit, cauliflower, and peanuts combat prostate cancer).
- Stabilizes blood sugar: artichokes, beans, garlic.
- Banishes bruises: cauliflower.
- Kills bacteria: mushrooms, onions, garlic, green tea.
- Saves eyesight: apricots, cantaloupe, carrots, broccoli, sweet potatoes, grapes, eggs, butterfat.
- Lowers cholesterol: artichokes, avocados, chestnuts, figs, beans, cantaloupe, onions, garlic, oats, walnuts, mushrooms, tomatoes, grapefruit, prunes, peanuts.
- Heals wounds: honey.
- Strengthens bones: bananas, beets, broccoli, cauliflower, pineapple, mushrooms, sweet potatoes.
- Promotes weight loss: figs, carrots, beets, cabbage, grapefruit, olive oil, peanuts, watermelon.
- Shields against Alzheimer's: apricots, mangoes, curcumin, coconut oil, salmon, sunflower seeds, eggs.
- Prevents constipation: apples, beans, cabbage, blueberries, peaches, prunes.
- Ends insomnia: cherries.
- Controls blood pressure: apricots, beets, cabbage, carrots, avocados, bananas, blueberries, chestnuts, mushrooms, garlic, lemons, limes, watermelon.
- Soothes sore throats: chili peppers.
- Quiets a cough: bananas.

- Helps hemorrhoids: beans, cabbage, peanuts.
- Guards against liver disease: artichokes.
- Clears sinuses: chili peppers.
- Smooths skin: lemons, limes, oats, olive oil, avocados.
- Cushions joints: apples.
- Fights allergies: honey.
- Conquers kidney stones: grapes, rice.
- Regulates thyroid: mangoes.
- Lifts mood: sweet potatoes.
- Fights fungus: garlic, onions.

This is just a short list of healing produce, but I think it shows there is enough natural help for our bodies without pharmaceutical drugs, which have side effects. These fruits and vegetables have no side effects. Please try to find fantastic recipes to use them in and discover a new way of life.

I learned to cook, first from my grandmother, and then my mother, then my mother-in-law, until I had quite a collection. I eat often and well and entertain often, cooking for friends and business associates... and have not had any complaints. I use most of the products I have listed here, but since I am not a vegan or a vegetarian, I add them to my beef, lamb, goat, chicken, and fish menus. With such a large selection, my meals have a great deal of variety, and my guests leave sated and happy.

Raw Milk
A Perfect Food

Like most Americans, I have believed all my life that the only safe, healthy milk was pasteurized!!!

WOW! Was I ever mistaken! Just like everything else I have learned from my research into nutrition these past three years, once again, the 'P.O.W.E.R.S.' that make money from misinformation have pulled the wool over our eyes.

The words of absolute truth I read from the Weston Price Foundation blew me away. "Raw whole milk from grass-fed cows is a complete and balanced food. You could literally live on it, and nothing else, for the rest of your life. Whole raw milk has both water and fat-soluble vitamins, completely available for your body to use. Nothing needs to be added to raw milk from grass-fed cows - no vitamins - no minerals - no enriching. It is a complete food."

I have resourced several well-known and respected sources for this article: the Weston Price Foundation, the largest U. S. non-profit organization, whose specific goal is the establishment of universal access to clean, certified raw milk; David Gumpert, author of *The Raw Milk Revolution*; Dr. Ron Schmid, a naturopathic physician who fought for the right of citizens to buy raw milk in Connecticut; Dr. Francis Potenger, President of the American Academy of Applied Nutrition in California; and Randolph Jonsson, nutrition consultant, Marin County, California.

In the early 1800's, cattle were kept adjacent to distilleries, being fed hot reeking swill left over from producing beer, wine, and whiskey. Sick cows created contaminated milk, a thin bluish white liquid. In the 1870's, Nathan Straus, a co-owner of Macy's, lost a child to diphtheria from that milk and promoted pasteurization throughout America and Europe. In 1889, Dr. Henry Coit also lost a child to contaminated swill milk, and in1893, formed the medical commission to certify clean milk production in New Jersey, enlisting dairy farmers to meet strict standards of production.

Pasteurization was invented at the same time dairy cows were being put out on farms to graze on pasture grasses. We mistakenly thought it was pasteurization that changed the health of milk. In 1944, when bogus magazine articles launched a smear campaign against raw milk, it added another faux level of condemnation.

Dr. Mercola states that government, public health officials, and the dairy industry officials restrict sales to control the market for factory farms.

Since there are no farms near me, I must bootleg milk. In order to buy raw milk in all but six states, you must go to the farm. You cannot buy it at farmer's markets or grocery stores or have it delivered to you. This is true here in Texas! I could easily buy drugs out on the street, but I have to seek out milk sources, hidden from anyone who cannot be trusted not to blow the whistle because the permit will be taken away from the dairy farmer!!!!!!!!

Bureaucrats and medical monopolists have stripped us of what should be an inalienable, constitutional right to purchase raw milk and other healthy, locally produced foods from the people who produce them. Today, there is a current yoke of prohibitions and bureaucratic red tape intended for commercial interests to control our food supply and thus, our health. Once again, follow the money!

It is truly sad, since raw milk is such a valuable, healing food; a powerful medicine with naturally occurring hormones and growth factors. Raw milk clears allergies; children's middle ear infections disappear and do not reappear.

Raw milk contains every known fat- and water-soluble vitamin: A, C, D, E, K, Bl, B2, B3 (Niacin), B6, Bl2, Pantothenic Acid, Biotin, Folic Acid. How amazing is that?

Vitamins must be added to pasteurized milk. Raw milk also contains a multitude of minerals:

Sodium, Potassium, Chloride, Iron, Zinc, Phosphorus, Magnesium, Copper, Manganese, Iodine, Selenium, Cobalt, Chromium, Molybdenum, Nickek, Silicon, Vanadium, and Calcium.

Calcium is an important element abundant in raw milk, promoting reduction of cancers, particularly of the colon, the formation of strong teeth and reduction of dental cavities, higher bone mineral density in every age grouping. It lowers the risk of kidney stones, osteoporosis, and fractures in older adults.

Minerals require a delicate balance with other minerals to function properly. (Calcium needs a proper ratio of phosphorus and magnesium). Nature codes the entire array of minerals in raw milk into a perfect balance.

Raw milk is the chief source of enzymes, a critical component in recovering from disease and establishing and maintaining health. There are sixty-plus enzymes essential in facilitating key reactions devoted to digestion and taking work off the pancreas. Amylase, lactase, lipase, and phosphatases break down starch, lactose (milk sugar), fat (triglycerides), and phosphate compounds, respectively, making milk more digestible and freeing up key minerals. Other enzymes: catalase, lysozyme, and lactoperoxidase help protect milk from unwanted bacterial infection, making it safer to drink.

These enzymes are killed by pasteurization heat.

Amino acids are the building blocks for protein (twenty to twenty-two are needed). Eight are essential and must be derived from food. The remaining twelve to fourteen are made in our cells from the essential eight.

Raw cow's milk has all eight essential amino acids. Eighty percent are caseins; they are heat stable, and easy to digest. Twenty percent are whey proteins, easy to digest, but heat sensitive. They are our antibiotic arsenal with important bioactivity. They include the anti-microbial activity of key enzymes, enzyme inhibitors, antibodies, metal binding proteins, vitamin binding proteins, and several growth factors.

Enzyme inhibitors break apart cell walls of undesirable bacteria and team up to knock out unwanted microbes. Antibodies provide resistance to many viruses, bacteria, and bacterial toxins; they also reduce the severity of asthma symptoms.

All of these disease fighters are lost when milk is heated to normal pasteurization temperature.

Two-thirds of the fat in raw milk is saturated. Saturated fats build cell membranes and key hormones and serve as a vehicle for important fat-soluble vitamins. They provide energy storage and padding for delicate organs. Fats cause our stomach lining to secrete a hormone to let us know when we've eaten enough. Non-fat dairy products and other fat free foods potentially contribute to over-eating.

Raw milk is the source of fat-soluble vitamins A and D. Contrary to popular opinion, liberal amounts of animal fats, particularly from grass-fed animals, are essential for good health and resistance to disease. Humans achieve perfect physical form and perfect health, generation after generation, only by consuming nutrient-dense whole foods and the vital fat-soluble activators found exclusively in animal fats.

This is true only for whole milk, not skim. By removing important fats and fat-soluble vitamins in the skimming process, the skim milk becomes a burden on the body, causing the liver to give up stored nutrients in order to digest it. The loss of CLA (conjugated linoleic acid), pathogen-busting medium-chain triglycerides and Vitamin A, alone constitutes an unforgivable crime against nature's perfect food.

CLA is a wonder fat. It offers eight great properties:

1. Muscle growth enhancement prevents muscle-wasting.
2. Inhibits fat formation, reduces abdominal body fat.
3. Improves insulin sensitivity.
4. Inhibits breast and prostate cancers.
5. Enhances immune system.
6. Lowers food allergy reactions.
7. Raises metabolic rate.
8. Lowers cholesterol/reduces cholesterol oxidation from meat and raw milk from grass-fed animals.

Grass-fed animals produce three to five times more CLA than grain-fed animals. Butterfat, the saturated fat in raw milk, absorbs and utilizes vitamins and minerals and antioxidants, nourishes our heart muscle, contains antifungal, anti-microbial, and anticancer agents, and is high in the all-important Omega-3 fatty acids (from Dr. Joseph Mercola's email newsletter).

Pasteurization (from a technique originally invented by French scientist Louis Pasteur for use on beer and wine) is a heating process designed to destroy all bacteria and most enzyme activity.

Homogenization forces whole milk through small orifices under very high pressure. It breaks down fat molecules and prevents cream from rising to the top. The intense pressure also subjects the milk to high heat a second time, altering color, flavor, and nutritional value.

Un-heated milk contains its full complement of enzymes and lactase-producing bacteria needed by our bodies to break down and assimilate the milk sugar, lactose. (These helpful bacteria are killed in the pasteurization/homogenization process). Chances are good that even if you have not been able to digest pasteurized milk, you will be able to drink raw milk, even if you are of African or Asian descent, who ethnically have had more problems with milk. Some may better tolerate fermented milk products, such as yogurt and kefir.

Cholesterol in raw milk is one of the body's repair substances... an antioxidant band-aid. If you eat artery-damaging foods such as hydrogenated and trans-fat laden vegetable oils, excess refined sugar, white flour, and over-cooked animal products, "good cholesterol" levels will rise in response to the assault, attempting to moderate the damage, according to Randolph Jonsson, nutrition consultant, Marin County, California.

Find the Weston A. Price raw milk web site, or just look up raw milk, and do some research yourself.

Seaweeds A Miracle for Beauty and Health

It was quite a surprise to me when I found out seaweed could promote beauty, as well as health for all of us. There are two different methods of use: in food preparation and in bathing.

You can crush, chop, snip, or crumble any dry sea green vegetables and mix them just as they are into soups, sauces, casseroles, rice, or noodles, and let them blend into your recipe. Roast them into pizzas, nachos, or focaccias. Pan toast them with Chinese noodles and ginger. If you like them in salads, remember that a vinegar dressing tenderizes sea greens just as cooking does. If you add sea greens, no other salt is needed. Sundried, they are convenient to buy, store, and use when you need them. Be sure to put them in a moisture-proof container, and they will keep indefinitely.

Seaweeds are a rich source of proteins, carbohydrates, minerals, amino acids, enzymes, fiber, antioxidants, and vitamins A, B,C, D, E, and K. They are one of the richest sources of iodine. Sea greens contain all fifty-six necessary trace elements for life, many of which have been depleted in the earth's soil. Sea greens protect us from heavy metals and radiation by-products, by converting them into harmless salts that our bodies can eliminate.

A seaweed bath is a great way to get the benefits of sea plants. Seaweed baths are Nature's perfect body-psyche balancer. Seaweed purifies and balances the ocean and performs many of the same functions for our bodies. Noticeable rejuvenating effects occur when toxins are released from your tissues. Sea greens are effective detoxifiers, strengthening us against disease and reducing excess stores of fluid and fat.

A seaweed soak is like a wet-steam sauna, only better, because sea greens balance body chemistry instead of dehydrating it. The electrolytic magnetic action of sea plants releases excess body fluids from congested cells and dissolves fatty wastes through skin, replacing them with key minerals. Vitamin K, a fat-soluble vitamin in seaweeds, aids adrenal activity, so a seaweed soak also helps maintain hormone balance for a more youthful body.

You can gather sea greens from the ocean if the waters are unpolluted. Do not take any that wash up on the shore, nor sea greens loose in the sea. They can harbor little bugs or mites that bite. Collect any that are still connected to the bottom, thus are still alive, using buckets or clean trash cans to take them home.

Run very hot water over the fresh or dried seaweed and fill so you will be covered completely when you lie down. The water will turn rich brown as the plants release their minerals. As you soak, the gel from the seaweed transfers onto your skin. This coating increases perspiration to release toxins from your system and replaces them by osmosis with minerals. Rub your skin, especially cellulite areas with the sea leaves during the bath to stimulate circulation, smooth and tone the body, and remove waste coming out on the skin surface.

When the sea greens have done their work, the gel coating dissolves and floats off the skin, and the leaves shrivel—a sign that the bath is over. Forty-five minutes is usually about right to balance the acid-alkaline system, and encourage liver activity, cellulite release, and fat metabolism. Skin tone, color, and better circulation are almost immediately noticeable. To get the most from a seaweed treatment, dry-brush cellulite areas before your seaweed bath to exfoliate dead skin and open pores for waste elimination and blood-flow to the affected area.

**Note: A seaweed soak is one of the most effective treatments in natural healing but use it with care. If you are under a doctor's care for heart disease or high blood pressure, check with your physician to see if a seaweed bath is okay for you.*

Sea greens are a beauty treatment. Seaweed adds amazing luster to the skin. Ancient sea-loving Greeks said that Aphrodite, the goddess of love who rose out of the foaming sea, owed her supple skin, shiny hair, and sparkling eyes to the plants of the sea. A seaweed face mask increases circulation, stimulates lymphatic drainage, and dilates capillaries to tone your skin. Applying seaweed can speed recovery from minor burns, clear acne, and heal scars.

Seaweed returns mineral salts to your skin that stress and pollution deplete. Skin cells hold moisture better when they absorb mineral salts, making the skin more supple and elastic. By retaining moisture, the skin plumps, removing the look of lines and wrinkles. Many women report smoother skin and better skin texture after a seaweed treatment. Amino acid, mineral, and vitamin content help nourish the skin, too. Some seaweeds possess molecules similar to collagen. (Collagen is the most abundant protein in our body. It is laced through every cell, organ, bone, and muscle and is the chief constituent of connective tissue for healthy skin, ligaments, and tendons.)

Here is a quick profile of sea plants—green, brown, red, and blue-green algae:

KELP (Laminaria), a brown sea plant containing vitamins A, B, D, E, and K, is a good source of vitamin C and is rich in minerals. Kelp proteins are comparable in quality to animal proteins. Kelp's sodium alginate (algin) helps remove radioactive particles and heavy metals from the body. Algin, carrageenan, and ager are kelp gels that rejuvenate gastrointestinal health. Kelp works as a blood purifier, relieves arthritis stiffness, and promotes adrenal, pituitary, and thyroid health. Kelp's iodine can normalize thyroid-related disorders like obesity and lymph system congestion. It is a demulcent that helps eliminate herpes outbreaks. Kelp is rich. A little goes a long way.

KOMBU (Laminaria digitata, setchelli, horsetail kelp) has a long tradition as a Japanese delicacy with great nutritional healing value. It is a decongestant for excess mucous and helps lower blood pressure. Kombu has abundant iodine, carotenes, B, C, D, and E vitamins, minerals such as calcium, magnesium, potassium, silica, iron, and zinc, and the powerful skin-healing nutrient, germanium. Kombu is a meaty, high-protein seaweed, higher in natural mineral salts than most other seaweeds. Add a strip of Kombu to your bean pot to reduce gas.

HIJIKI (Hizikia fusiforme) is a mineral-rich, high-fiber seaweed, with 20% protein, vitamin A, carotenes, and calcium. Hijiki has the most calcium of any sea green, 1400 mg per 100 grams of dry weight. Japanese studies reveal Hijiki boosts natural killer T-cells for more disease protection.

NORI (Porphyra, Laver) is a red sea plant with a sweet meaty taste when dried. It contains nearly 50% balanced protein, higher than any other sea plant. Tests find that protein and carbohydrates from Japanese Nori are 70% assimilable, very high for a vegetable. Nori's fiber makes it a perfect sushi wrapper. Nori is rich in all the carotenes, calcium, iodine, iron, and phosphorus.

ARAME (Eisenia bycyclis) is one of the ocean's richest sources of iodine. Herbalists use Arame to help reduce breast and uterine fibroids, and through its fat-soluble vitamins and phytohormones, to normalize menopausal symptoms. Arame promotes soft, wrinkle-free skin, enhances hair's glossiness, and prevents hair loss.

SEA PALM (Postelsia palmaeformis), American Arame, grows only on the Pacific Coast of North America. One of my favorites, it has a sweet, salty taste that goes especially well as a vegetable, rice, or salad topping.

BLADDERWRACK (Fucus vesiculosus) is packed with vitamin K, an excellent adrenal stimulant. It is still used today by native Americans in steam baths for arthritis, gout, and illness recovery.

WAKAME (Alaria, Undaria) is a high-protein, high calcium seaweed, with carotenes, iron and vitamin C. Widely used in the Orient for hair growth and luster and for skin tone.

DULSE (Palmaria palmate), a red sea plant, is rich in iron, protein, and vitamin A. It is a supremely balanced nutrient, with 300 times more iodine and 50 times more iron than wheat. Tests of Dulse show activity against the herpes virus. It has purifying and tonic effects on the body, yet its natural balanced salts nourish as a mineral, without inducing thirst.

IRISH MOSS (Chondrus crispus, Sarrageen) is full of electrolyte minerals: calcium, magnesium, sodium, and potassium. Its mucilaginous compounds help you detoxify, boost metabolism, and strengthen hair, skin, and nails. It is traditionally used for low sex drive.

I don't think Americans know much about the marvelous qualities of sea greens. Please read this column with a great deal of concentration. The knowledge I gained in researching this topic surprised me as much as I think it will surprise most of you.

Sea vegetables can solve many of the aches, pains, and illnesses that we have with a minimum of monetary output and an easy way to obtain them. I am going to the Oriental grocery in Austin this week to expedite this new (to me) source of nutrition and healing. Hope you do the same.

Minerals

Sea greens help re-mineralize us.
Sea greens contain all the necessary
trace elements for life, many of which
are depleted in the earth's soil.
They are powerful healers.
They are the most nutritionally dense plants
on the planet.

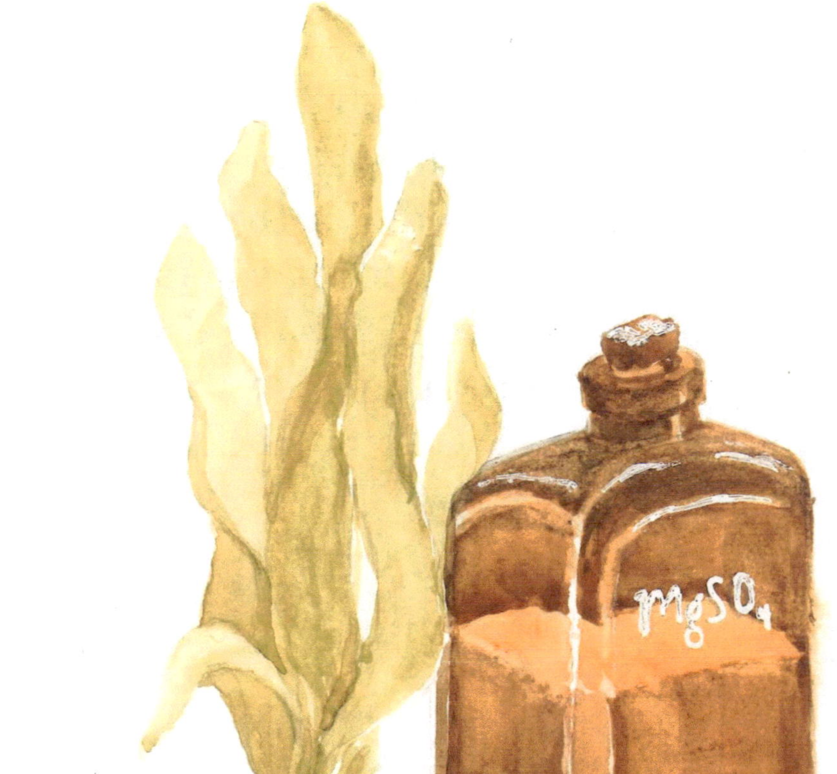
MgSO4

Iodine and the Thyroid

It is amazing how iodine and thyroid interconnect. Did you know that iodine is responsible for all the hormones in the body? It has anti-bacterial, anti-viral, anti-parasitic, and anti-cancer properties (Dr. David Brownstein). A deficiency of iodine is a major cause of hypothyroidism, or under-activity, of the thyroid gland. In 1940, our American diet contained 500-800 mcg. of iodine. By 1995, it had dropped to 135 mcg.

Fluoride, bromine, and chlorine are all *halogens* and interfere with thyroid function. They have similar chemical properties as iodine and attach to the same receptors in your cells, competing with iodine. Food manufacturers have stopped using iodine in baked goods and are using bromine instead. Our water supply contains chlorine and fluoride. So, they also compete with iodine to get into your cells. And you cannot avoid chlorine and fluoride simply by drinking filtered water. You get a hefty dose any time you bathe, shower, soak in a hot tub, or swim in a swimming pool. Fluoride is also in almost all toothpastes and mouthwashes. Bromine is in some pesticides (another good reason for buying organic food with no pesticides). We need more iodine to compete with these disruptors.

Dr. Nan Katherine Fuchs, a medical doctor who specializes in nutritional medicine, says, "Most conventional doctors never test for iodine deficiency. They figure there is no need to test iodine levels when they can just test your thyroid function instead. The problem with this is that the most widely used thyroid test, TSH (thyroid stimulating hormone) is wildly inaccurate. While the TSH measures thyroid hormone, it cannot tell the difference between *active thyroid hormone with iodine, and de-activated thyroid hormone with bromine or chlorine or fluorine!*"

Dr. Andrew Weil states, "Unfortunately, thyroid function tests are not reliable, sometimes indicating that people are in normal thyroid balance when they are not."

Dr. Julian Whitaker says, "Laboratory blood tests will definitely pick up on severe thyroid-deficiency states. The mild hypothyroidism that many people experience does not register on these sophisticated tests. This leads many physicians to believe the symptoms are merely 'in the head' of the patient."

Signs of hypothyroidism are dry skin, brittle hair, constipation, feeling cold, chronic fatigue, depression, weight gain, muscle and joint stiffness, and headaches. The individual's metabolic processes slow down. Thyroid hormones regulate metabolism in every cell.

Hyperthyroidism or "Graves' Disease" is an overactive metabolism, where too much thyroid is being produced, causing weight loss, rapid heartbeat, climate sensitivity (feeling hot), bulging eyes, blurred vision, nervous tension, irritability, sweating and tremors, itching, diarrhea, arthritis-like swelling of joints, and, caused by stress, overuse of diet pills, mental burnout, and fatigue. A different approach to treatment is used for hypothyroidism.

Doctors use two different treatments for hypothyroidism. One is "Synthroid," a synthetic. The other, "Armour," is a natural desiccated thyroid. Dr. William Campbell Douglass says, "Synthroid, the synthetic thyroid, produces two hormones: 99.97% T4 (thyroxine), and .1% T3 (triiodothyronine). The body must convert T4 to T3 to control metabolism. Many patients do not have the enzymatic capability to make that conversion, so taking Synthroid is an exercise in futility."

He switched patients to Armour, a natural thyroid product; a combination of T3 and T4. The majority of these patients experienced an almost immediate improvement.

Dr. Whitaker stated that desiccated natural thyroid contains a range of thyroid hormones; synthetic hormones are more limited.

Dr. Linda Page, a naturopathic physician, said synthetic thyroid drugs are linked to bone loss, headaches, insomnia, and tachycardia. She also suggested that to simulate the thyroid, press the hollow at the base of the throat, three times for ten seconds each.

Dr. Weil warns against attempting to stop Synthroid suddenly. You should experiment cutting down dosage very gradually, giving yourself a few weeks at each new level to see how you feel.

Dr. Campbell says soy contains the isoflavone genistein, a powerful anti-thyroid agent, suppressing thyroid function. Soy, as a phytoestrogen, acts like a hormone and can easily throw off the delicate balance of the thyroid hormonal system.

Dr. Page says thyroid function can be hampered by an iodine deficiency from x-rays or low dose radiation (mammograms), excessive dieting, or soy.

The best nutrients for thyroid health are iodine and potassium, found in rich sea greens. Ounce for ounce, along with herbs, sea greens are higher in vitamins and minerals than any other food. Sea plants come in green, brown, red, and blue-green algae. Some of these are Dulse, Nori, Irish moss, Kelp, Kombu, Hijiki, Wakame, Arame, and Focus (Bladderwrack).

Sea greens help re-mineralize us. Sea greens contain all the necessary trace elements for life, many of which are depleted in the earth's soil. They are powerful healers. They are the most nutritionally dense plants on the planet.

In our era of processed foods and iodine-poor soils, sea greens and sea foods stand alone as potent sources of natural, balanced iodine. Iodine is essential to life. The thyroid gland cannot make thyroxine, the enzyme that regulates metabolism, without it. Iodine is an important element of alertness, rapid brain activity, and a prime deterrent to arterial plaque.

Thyroid hormones are created from iodine and the amino acid tyrosine. Thyro-Globulin, the mixture of tyrosine and iodine stored in the thyroid gland, is transformed into hormones that regulate our metabolism, protein, carbohydrate, carotene use, and cholesterol (sea greens help lower cholesterol). Along with the adrenal glands, the amount of thyroid hormone released into the bloodstream determines the body's base energy level. Sea plants nourish an underactive thyroid and normalize adrenal functions to trigger increased libido.

Preventive measures may be taken against iodine deficiency by adding just two tablespoons of chopped, dried sea greens to your daily diet.

A seaweed bath is a great way to get the benefits of sea plants. Seaweed baths are Nature's perfect body balancer.

To find a physician able to assist you with natural thyroid treatments:

American College for Advancement in Medicine,
www.acam.org (800) 532-3688

American Association of Naturopathic Physicians,
www.naturopathic.org.

Is Salt Necessary?

We have been told over and over again by doctors (and the media): "Don't eat salt! It will cause a heart attack!" ...but they do not stipulate what kind of salt.

Processed salt is dead, a toxin contributing to imbalance, which the immune system has to work to expel. Processed salt is bleached, heated, kiln-dried, and altered with pollutants and chemicals (such as chlorine).

We have been calling this salt, "Table Salt." Table salt is highly refined; a product of chemical and high-temperature industrial processes that remove all the valuable magnesium salts, as well as trace minerals naturally occurring in sea salt.

Refiners adulterate sea salt with several harmful additives, including aluminum compounds to replace natural iodine salts removed during processing. Potassium iodide is added in amounts that can be toxic. To stabilize the volatile iodide compound, dextrose is added, turning salt purple. Then a bleaching agent is necessary to restore whiteness.

"Table Salt, chemically treated, will no longer combine with human body fluid, invariably causing severe problems of edema (water retention) and other health disturbances." (Jacques DeLangre, "Seasalt's Hidden Powers.")

It is a myth that table salt is the major source of sodium in our diets. The truth is that we consume 10% in our food, 15% in the salt we add, and 75% is added by grocery food-processing, and from antacids, laxatives, sleeping pills, and over-the-counter aids. Fat-free foods (mayonnaise, margarine, soups, cream cheese, etc.) double their salt content to make up for their lack of taste. The average American consumes 8,000 to 10,000 mg. per day. (Linda Page, "Healthy Healing," 12th Edition.)

Table salt is 99.9% pure sodium chloride. Sea salt is 95% sodium chloride + 4% potassium chloride + 1% of eighty-four ionically-charged minerals and trace elements.

Sea salt is obtained from a salt dome or from the sea, not processed, not refined... nothing added. Sea salt is good for us. We should have one teaspoon of salt a day. It balances our potassium, magnesium, and calcium, while relaxing muscles, increasing circulation, and reducing fluid retention. It boosts our immune system. It also increases absorption of essential nutrients.

Sea salt and heavy water consumption is what one cutting-edge doctor uses to cure high blood pressure.

Sodium is a necessary nutrient to human existence. Naturally-occurring sodium, accompanied by its partner-mineral, potassium, regulates blood pressure, transmits nerve impulses, and maintains muscle activity. Together, sodium and potassium pump nutrients into the cells to nourish them and drain waste-products out to clean them. The sodium/potassium relationship also helps maintain fluid balance, so excess fluid or dehydration does not occur. Sodium is necessary for muscle contraction. Without sodium, the body cannot use calcium. Sodium keeps glands and organs healthy.

"Salt plays an essential role in digestion, starting from the moment food enters your mouth. Salt activates the primary digestive enzyme in the mouth, salivary amylase. Farther down the digestive tract, in the stomach, sodium chloride generates hydrochloric acid in the cells of the stomach wall, an essential secretion for proper digestion. Vegetarians have been led to believe that veggies provide all the salt they need in their diet. This is completely false. Why then are salt blocks provided for grazing animals? Because every farmer knows that without it, his vegetarian animals will get sick.

"Salt is the single element required for proper breakdown of plant carbohydrates into usable and assimilable human food. A salt-free, vegetarian diet is a sure ticket to the hospital and premature old age. Vegetarians are also prone to sugar addiction. The physiological explanation for this is that glucosides in grains are not digested without the presence of salt. As the body is denied these natural sugars, a deficiency develops and there is an insatiable desire to eat sweets." (Dr. Wm. C. Douglass, "Second Opinion.")

Dr. Peter Glidden, a very well-respected naturopathic doctor for two generations, teaching "Wholistic" Health, said about sea salt, "Your body gets the chloride ion it needs to keep the stomach acid strong and healthy. If you don't have enough salt, your stomach acid will be weak. If your stomach acid is weak, you cannot digest your food completely. If you cannot digest your food completely, you develop nutrient deficiencies. Nutrient deficiencies are the MAIN CAUSE of all chronic disease. Heartburn is caused by not enough stomach acid. Start salting your food, and your heartburn will disappear in about 3 weeks.

"The fear of salt today and the virtual ban on consuming products with high sodium content is a serious concern to biologists. Salt-free diets can cause salt starvation, which is a starvation of macro-and trace minerals, a biological deficiency that refined sodium chloride alone cannot correct. Too little sodium leads to low vitality, stagnant blood, and loss of clear thinking, because the brain depends on good fluid circulation."

Salt deficiency leads to loss of taste, cramps, weakness, lassitude, and severe cardio distress upon exertion.

Diuretics, excessive sweating, fever, diarrhea, heat, and too much exercise can cause severe sodium imbalance, and make the body lose too much salt.

If you crave salt, you may be lacking in chlorides, sodium, and iodine, which can be derived from fish, raw goat milk, and sea vegetables, or you may be lacking in zinc. (And you probably have not been using sea salt.)

The Daily use of natural sea salt bolsters thyroid function. The proper way to take in minerals is through the use of unrefined sea salt. There are a variety of everyday uses for salt:

- moisten and rub salt on bee sting to ease them.
- gargle warm water and salt for a sore throat.
- ½ teaspoon of salt in a pint of water will reduce tired and puffy eyes.
- rub salt and oil on skin to exfoliate it and stimulate lymph glands.
- add a pinch to water to lengthen flower life.
- for bath salts, add two ounces of sea salt to three droppers of an essential oil.
- spray with three tablespoons salt to one gallon water to kill poison ivy plant.
- remove table ring on wooden table by rubbing on salad oil and salt and letting stand one hour.
- rub in cups to remove tea or coffee stains.
- soak vases in brine if you cannot reach to scrub.
- deodorize a thermos or jug.
- rub on tarnished silver before washing.
- rub on eggy dishes for easy clean-up.
- rix with lemon juice to remove mildew.
- remove onion odor on your hands.
- remove stains on pots.
- rub on wine stains, let dry, rinse in cold water.
- clean, deodorize and sanitize your homeby combining salt with

lemon juice or vinegar and baking soda.
- starting at four months, give babies one yolk a day to supply cholesterol needed for mental development. Adding a pinch of sea salt to the yolk will also facilitate brain development.

Salt is necessary to activate the formulation of glial cells in the brain that make connections and help us think faster. Unfortunately, salt is often left out of commercial baby food, in the mistaken belief that salt should be avoided.

Does all this amaze you? After all we have heard to the contrary. Wow! It *did* surprise me before I started researching salt.

Magnificent Magnesium

Magnesium is responsible for over 300 biochemical reactions in your body.

Magnesium is the fourth most abundant mineral in the body, but 72% of Americans are deficient in magnesium (magnesium deficiency is worldwide). 50% of total body magnesium is found in the bones.

Magnesium

- is nature's Valium.
- helps muscles to relax; calcium causes them to contract.
- prevents calcium from building up in your arteries.
- activates enzymes, contributing to energy production, and helps regulate vitamin and mineral levels necessary to restore noise-related hearing loss.
- is a critical mineral for skeletal structure and is important for tooth formation.
- is necessary for good nerve and muscle function and athletic endurance.
- is also critical for heart vessel health and balanced blood pressure, and aids the heart and kidneys.
- aids in regulating heartbeat.
- counteracts stress, depression, and emotional instability, and brings

about restful sleep.
- aids the body's detoxification processes, helping prevent damage from environmental chemicals, heavy metals, and other toxins.
- helps the regulation of blood sugar levels.
- eases breathing for asthma sufferers.
- keeps muscles flexible and prevents cramps.
- Children with ADHD are found to be deficient in magnesium, as are diabetics.

Vitamin D3, vitamin K2, and calcium work together with magnesium.

A lack of magnesium can cause constipation, migraines, lack of sleep, anxiety, lack of appetite, numbness and tingling, fatigue and weakness, alcoholism, muscle contractions and cramps, asthma, osteoporosis, tooth decay, pregnancy problems, PMS, kidney stones, hypoglycemia, eye twitches, blood clots, abnormal heart rhythms, fibromyalgia, chronic neck and back pain, vertigo, and confusion.

Overconsumption of processed foods is usually a culprit in magnesium deficiency.

The following drugs steal magnesium from your body and cause deficiency:

- Diuretics for water retention or high blood pressure
- Lasix (Furosemide)
- Butex (Bumetanide)
- Thiaside
- Edecrin (ethacrynic acid)
- Metformin (Metformin/glucophage)
- Proton Pump Inhibitor (PPI) to treat acid reflux and gastritis, because the stomach acid being suppressed is required to absorb magnesium (Nexium, Prevacid).

Since the 1950s when synthetic fertilizer became prominent, our soil has been depleted of magnesium. It takes organic compost and manure to give us nutritious vegetables.

You must eat foods that contain magnesium, or supplements will not work alone. Sea vegetables, fish, poultry, dairy foods, green leafy vegetables, berries, seeds, nuts, cocoa, beans, fruits, avocados, garlic, parsley, asparagus, peas with skins, cucurbits, dried herbs and spices (coriander, dill, sage, basil), and flaxseed all carry magnesium.

Transdermal magnesium chloride spray is absorbed through the skin and it quickly goes wherever it is needed in the body. (Mix three ounces of magnesium chloride oil with one quart of water to make spray). When we take magnesium capsules, some of it is lost in our digestive function. The spray is completely absorbed. You can rub oil spray on painful areas to help stop the pain. If you get a cramp, spray that area. Our "herb lady" JoAnne Boudreau suggested spraying your children after a bedtime bath, and they will sleep better and do better in school on the morrow.

The dosage of magnesium capsules is 500 to 600 mg a day. I take magnesium capsules each day, and at night I spray with the oil. I would not be without magnesium supplementation.

Zinc: A Most Important Element!

Zinc is the cornerstone of our immune system and is absolutely necessary for growth and development. Zinc promotes immune system health and cellular repair and is a major constituent of wound recovery and healing.

Zinc:

- is a multipurpose antioxidant and has anti-viral activity, aiding brain function and lessening excitotoxicity (which damages our neurons). Zinc is a brain food that helps control mental disorders and promotes mental alertness.
- has almost been exhausted in our soil. And it has almost been destroyed by commercial food processing.

Stress depletes zinc, impairing the body's ability to heal. Little sleep, long hours, and injury recovery all require us to add more zinc to replace that which has been lost.

Zinc

- protects against free-radical damage; is essential for gland and sexual reproductive health; and is a key element in testosterone production, restoring a healthy balance of testosterone. The prostate gland contains more zinc than any other organ, thus strengthening the prostate and increasing low sperm count.

- is a detoxifier, protecting against mercury, cadmium, and other metals. High zinc concentrations reside in bone, skin, kidney, liver, pancreas, the retina, and prostate gland; and is primarily stored in muscle (65%) and red and white blood cells. Zinc is needed for proper bone formation and mineral uptake, and benefits patients with chronic pancreatitis.
- is more concentrated in the macula of the eye than anywhere else (except for the prostate and hearing organs), and zinc and selenium are used intravenously by cutting-edge doctors in correcting macular degeneration. Those with cataracts are low in zinc, as are those with night-blindness. Zinc is crucial for eye health.
- strengthens the GI tract and helps repair gut cells in inflammatory bowel disease.
- protects the thymus and lymphoid tissues, aids the thyroid gland, and reduces the duration of colds. Zinc lozenges are of primary help here.
- increases HDL cholesterol and decreases LDL. Zinc's antioxidant prevents LDL cholesterol from converting into 'little l(pa) lipoprotein' plaque! Zinc can cure angina in fourteen days with a special format protocol.

White spots on fingernails correlate with low zinc, as well as dry skin, hair loss, and acne (zinc metabolizes fatty acids). Zinc helps reduce diabetes in women. Alzheimer's patients are deficient in zinc. Obese children are deficient.

Inadequate zinc levels cause chronic pain. It is important that all of us take 30 mg of zinc per day, regardless of our age, twenty, thirty, forty, fifty, and over. Adequate levels reduce the risk of infection, flu, diabetes, obesity, glucose tolerance, and release of insulin.

Protein is the main source of zinc in our diets, so vegetarians can run short, unless they find an alternative source such as some nuts and sea vegetables. Breads, cereals, and legumes bind plant sources of zinc and prevent the body from using it.

Dietary zinc:

- oysters 74%
- chuck roast 7%

- lobster 3.4%
- pork loin 2.9%
- baked beans 2.9%
- chicken 2.4%
- yogurt 1.7%
- cashews 1.6%

Now, if that isn't enough to cause us to beef up on zinc, we find a problem called immuno-senescence, which is the aging of the immune system. As we age, we lose zinc. This causes a majority of our elders (sixty and older) to be deficient in zinc, which contributes to atherosclerosis, cancer, osteoporosis, neurological disorders, excessive sweat, and autoimmune diseases - where the immune system attacks and destroys healthy body tissue, like lupus and rheumatoid arthritis.

Now it figures broadly in international health programs aimed at reducing death tolls from diseases such as severe diarrhea, malaria, pneumonia, and tuberculosis.

(Originally published in July 2014)

Herbs

PEPPERMINT:
Peppermint tea helps soothe the stomach lining and fend off nausea and vomiting; encourages digestion by stimulating the gallbladder and liver, especially after a fatty meal; relieves flu symptoms; stops hiccups.

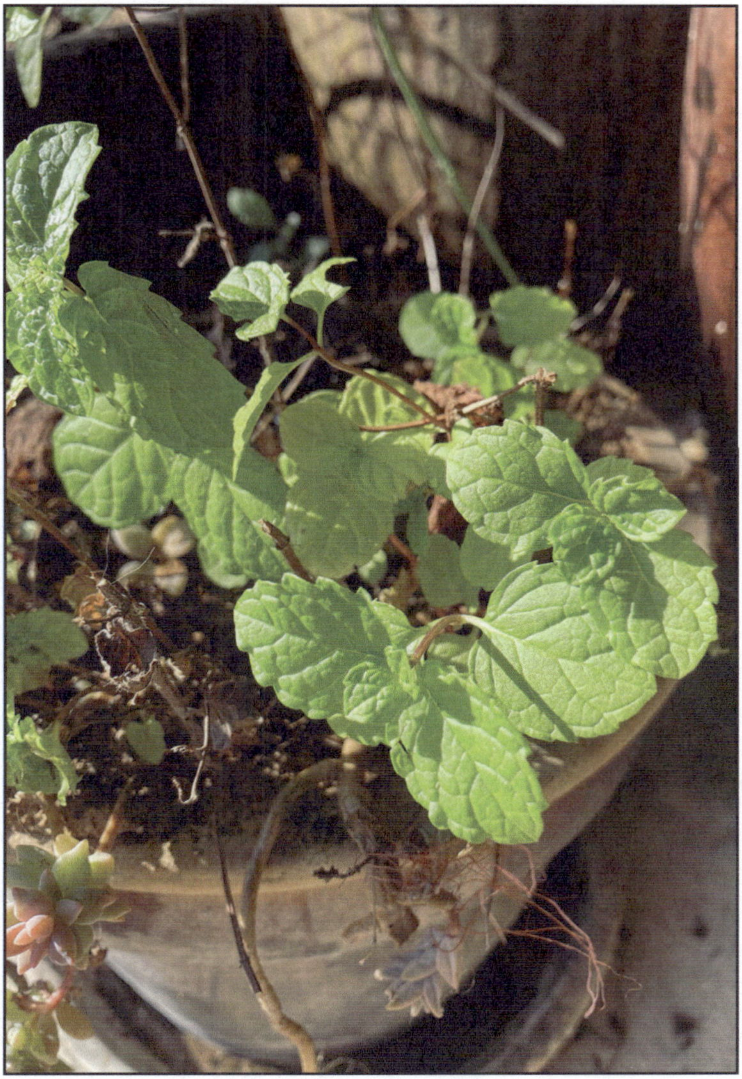

A Shocking Revelation!

HERBS, Nature's Gift That Counteracts and Prevents Disease

I thought that you, my readers, might like to have a written list of healing herbs and their properties that you may or may not even have heard of. Duplicate this on your home copier or at a commercial copier's.

- OLIVE LEAF: Greatest antibiotic for viral, bacterial, and fungal diseases. Protects against staph, poliovirus, anthrax, and AIDS.
- HORSETAIL TEA: Antiseptic properties cleanse and heal kidney, bladder, and prostate. Dissolves stones, repairs hernia (six months), strengthens hair, nails, tooth enamel. (Anger, fear, resentment, and depression affect kidneys and bladder).
- FLAX SEED: (Instead of chemo) Treats allergies, high blood pressure, acne, eczema, psoriasis, breast lumps, MS, ADD, arthritis, depression, immune disorder, eye/heart/joint problems, high cholesterol. Lubricates dry, flaky scalp and skin, colon.

MENTAL HEALTH, NERVOUS SYSTEM

- BUTTERBUR: Migraines, 100 mg; anti-inflammatory; seasonal allergies, 50-75 mg 2x per day. *Must be labeled "PA free." do not use while pregnant or nursing.
- FEVERFEW: Migraines: chew leaf. Anti-inflammatory. Magnesium, vitamin B2 and feverfew are a good combination. *Do not use while pregnant.
- HOPS: nervousness, insomnia, menopause/hot flashes, digestion, relieves toothache, nerve pain. Tea or capsules, 500 mg 1-3x per day.
- KAVA (root): anxiety, menopause. Water solvent, not alcohol. *Do not take with liver problems. Do not take with prescription medicines or aspirin, Tylenol, Motrin, etc.

- LEMON BALM (leaves): anxiety, stress, colic, digestion, fever blisters.
- PASSION FLOWER (flower, leaves, stems, root): anxiety, insomnia. *May interfere with blood thinning medication. Do not use while pregnant.
- ST. JOHN'S WORT (dried flowers): minor depression, muscle aches, fever blisters, PMS. *Herb/drugs interaction.
- VALERIAN (roots): nervousness, insomnia, anxiety. Not habit forming.

RESPIRATORY

- ASTRAGALUS (roots): immune support, viral infections, tonic. Prevents colds,flu.
- ECHINACEA (leaves, stems, roots): boosts immune system, colds and flu, wounds. *Herb/drugs interaction.
- ELDER (flowers, fruits): respiratory system.
- EUCALYPTUS (leaves, oil… in tea or capsules): colds, cough, asthma, emphysema. *Herb/drugs interaction… may cause low blood sugar. Caution diabetics.
- LICORICE (rhysomes): antiviral and antibacterial, sore throat, cough, heartburn, gastritis, stomach ulcers, soothes irritated mucous membranes. Lozenges, tea.
- MULLEIN (leaves, flowers; NOT seeds) ear infections, respiratory.
- PELARGONIUM (geranium roots): bronchitis, colds and flu, sinusitis. Lozenges and tinctures.
- SAGE (salvia): sore throat, colds, coughs, memory and cognition, GI tract, menopause/excessive sweating, hot flashes, and night sweats.
- THYME (leaves, flowers, oil): respiratory, digestive system.

HEART AND CIRCULATION

- BILBERRY (leaves and fruits): potent antioxidant, diarrhea, circulation, varicose veins, eye health, atherosclerosis.
- CACAO (chocolate): anti-inflammatory, flavonoid antioxidants, beneficial cardiovascular effects, lowers blood pressure, slows blood clotting (similar to aspirin), lowers LDL oxidation, increases HDL. May increase the chance of surviving a heart attack.
- CINNAMON: diabetes, digestion, treatment for colds, flu, coughs,

chest infections. Increases blood flow to hands and feet.

- GINKGO: improves blood flow to brain; helps treat dementia and Alzheimer's, tinnitus, macular degeneration, intermittent claudication (cramping and pain caused by poor blood flow in legs); contains potent antioxidants to protect nerve cells and terpene lactones which reduce inflammation. *Do not use during pregnancy.
- GRAPES, GRAPE SEED: rich in antioxidants, lowers high cholesterol and blood pressure, aids circulatory ailments including coronary heart disease, chronic venous insufficiency, varicose veins. Regulates blood sugar levels, relieves asthma allergies, treats eye disorders.
- HAWTHORN (leaves, flowers, fruits): treats mild congestive heart failure, minor heart arrhythmias, strengthens force of heart muscle, maintains normal heart rhythm and healthy blood pressure. Antioxidant, helps protect cells from damage.
- HIBISCUS (fruits, leaves): Diuretic and mild laxative, treats colds, coughs, heart disorders. Loaded with vitamin C and mucilage, pectin, anthocyanins (antioxidants that protect cell membranes, soothing irritated tissues of mouth, throat, and gastric tract). Exerts beneficial effects on blood pressure and cholesterol, weight loss. Reduces blood pressure to same degree as two prescriptions: Captopril and Lisinopril.
- HORSE CHESTNUT (flowers, leaves, bark, seeds): Improves varicose veins, hemorrhoids, chronic venous insufficiency, swelling ankles; relieves nighttime leg cramping, pain, and itching, reduces swelling and tenderness after injury.
- RESVERTROL (Grapes, Grape Seed) (skins, seeds, stems): rich in antioxidants, lowers high cholesterol and blood pressure, aid circulatory ailments-including coronary heart disease, chronic venous insufficiency, varicose veins; regulates blood sugar levels, relieves asthma and allergies, treats eye disorders.
- TEA (leaves, buds; mainly green tea): heart health, cholesterol, anti-inflammatory, antioxidant, weight loss, cancer prevention.

DIGESTIVE SYSTEM

- CHAMOMILE (dried flowers, oil): Aids digestion and inflammation, heartburn, flatulence, diarrhea, infant colic, gastritis, Crohn's disease, irritable bowel syndrome. Relieves muscle tension, eases anxiety, soothes irritated or inflamed skin and eczema. As a mouthwash, prevents mouth sores from chemo and radiation.

- FENNEL (all parts edible; seeds, tea): Digestion, bloating, gas, diarrhea, upset stomach, menstrual cramps. Improves appetite, reduces food cravings, buffers cramping from laxatives, increases breast milk, freshens breath, thins mucus, aids expectoration. Gargle for coughs and sore throats.
- GARLIC (cloves): Antibiotic, decreases infections in gut and lungs, diarrhea, improves heart health, prostate cancer, lowers cholesterol and blood pressure, reduces blood clots, strengthens immunity.
- GINGER (roots): Digestive tract, soothes nausea. Effective against colds, flu, sore throat, headaches, menstruation, colitis, arthritis.
- GOLDENSEAL (roots): Digestion, diarrhea, antimicrobial, peptic ulcers, psoriasis, mouth ulcers. Contains berberine; destroys Giardia.
- MILK THISTLE/Silymarin (seeds, all parts edible): protects liver, including against acetaminophen-caused liver damage, viral hepatitis, liver cirrhosis, chronic liver disease, gallbladder, antidote for mushroom poisoning. (Absorption enhanced with Phosphatidyl choline).
- PEPPERMINT (leaves, oil): indigestion, IBS, colds, coughs, muscle aches, tension headache, bug bite itching. Do not take with GERD or hiatal hernia.
- PSYLLIUM (seeds and husks): bulk laxative, fiber, heart health, cholesterol lowering, blood pressure, weight control.
- SLIPPERY ELM (bark, wood): heartburn, coughs, sore throat, itchy inflamed skin, stomach, intestines, GERD, Crohn's disease, heals inflamed mucosal tissue.
- TURMERIC/Curcumin (roots): digestion and liver problems, joint pain, skin conditions, kills/reduces cancer cells, diarrhea, may offer protection from Alzheimer's plaque. May prevent every common disease.

This is a lot to absorb at one time. You may have to read it a few times, and then decide which herb or herbs to use for your particular problems.

Many of you are not aware of the efficacy of herbs, but they have been used for centuries… long before pharmaceutical drugs were around. Indigenous peoples have been using herbs for healing for thousands of years.

I will continue with more information next month on these valuable gifts from nature.

Healing Herbs

(Part Two)

When I discovered a well-known, respected, factual book on herbs (a subject most of us know little about), I decided to expand my readers' knowledge along with mine. We have become aware of vitamins and minerals… even enzymes and amino acids… in our quest for healthy bodies and minds in the past ten years or so, but herbal information has not been in the limelight. We think of it as "Eastern Medicine," not as readily in our sphere. I was surprised at the immense healing ability of simple plants, a number of which we can plant and raise ourselves.

This will continue the categories of healing herbs that began in last month's article.

JOINTS, MUSCLES, SKIN

- ALOE (mucilaginous, gooey gel): Antibacterial. Burns, cuts, colitis 25-30 mg (2 tbsp), 2x per day; psoriasis, diabetes 10-20 mg (1 tbsp) daily.
- ARNICA MONTANA (flowers and leaves): Use gel for arthritis and rheumatic pain, phlebitis, swelling due to fractures, acne, chapped lips; to ease pain of sore muscles, bruises, sprains. *Do not take internally or use on broken skin.
- CALENDULA (edible flowers): Antioxidant, anti-inflammatory. Heals skin ailments, acne, eczema, wounds, and fights gum inflammation.
- CAT'S CLAW (bark, roots): Asthma, arthritis, rheumatism, urinary tract, kidney problems, cancer, intestinal ailments,

gonorrhea, a form of birth control, inflammation, joint problems, gastritis, ulcers, neuralgia, HIV, immune system booster, protection against NSAIDs (e.g., ibuprofen). *Do not take if pregnant or nursing. Not for children under three years of age.

- CAYENNE (fruits): Apply topically for arthritis, nerve pain, shingles, itching and inflammation of psoriasis. Taken internally, may reduce blood cholesterol and triglycerides, cluster headaches, improve circulation, relieve heartburn, stimulate stomach lining cells. and prevent ulcers, help regulate blood sugar levels.
- COMFREY (leaves, roots): Anti-inflammatory and analgesic. Joint pain, heal sprains, bruises and minor wounds, mend broken bones, relieve upper or lower back pain. *Use only topical preparations, relieved of the pyrrolizidine alkaloids… could hurt liver otherwise.
- DEVIL'S CLAW (roots): Anti-inflammatory. Arthritis, back pain, headaches, fibromyalgia, lowers fever, stimulates digestion.
- ROSEMARY (leaves, twigs): Antimicrobial, antioxidant, antibacterial. Topically… Muscle and joint pain, bronchitis, circulation, memory/cognition. Internally… Indigestion, headache, nervous tension.Aromatherapy… Stress and anxiety.
- TEA TREE OIL: Antiseptic. Effective against antibiotic-resistant bacteria MRSA (methicillin resistant staphylococcus aureas), herpes virus, fungal and bacterial skin infections, gingivitis, dandruff, acne.
- WILLOW BARK: Headache, back pain, fever, osteoarthritis, sprains, cold and flu, toothache. Takes the place of aspirin.

URINARY AND MALE HEALTH

- JUNIPER (berries): Urinary tract infections, bronchitis, respiratory conditions.
- PARSLEY (leaves, roots, seeds): Anti-inflammatory, diuretic, circulatory. Urinary tract infections, kidney stones, high blood pressure, calms indigestion, helps stimulate normal menstruation. *Do not take with blood pressure meds… lowers blood pressure.
- POMEGRANATE (fruit and seeds): Antioxidant with strong protection against atherosclerosis, prostate cancer. Promotes circulatory system health.
- PYGEUM (bark): Anti-inflammatory. Bladder pain, urinary tract, malaria, fever, lung ailments, stomach and intestinal disorders,

kidney disease, infertility, BPH (benign prostatic hyperplasia), menstrual complaints.

- SAW PALMETTO (fruits and berries): Benign prostatic hyperplasia (BPH), Urinary tract infections, chronic pelvic pain, bladder disorders, gallbladder problems.
- STINGING NETTLE (leaves, roots): Benign prostatic hyperplasia (BPH), Arthritis, allergies, diuretic, urinary tract infection, chronic skin problems, psoriasis, tendonitis, sprains, strains. Can interfere with medicines for diabetes, high blood pressure, anxiety, insomnia.
- TOMATO: Antioxidant, prostatic cancer prevention.
- UVA URSI (bearberry): (leaves) Anti-bacterial. Urinary tract infections. *Not for nursing mothers, pregnancy, children, renal failure.
-

FEMALE HEALTH

- BLACK COHOSH (roots, rhizomes): Premenstrual syndrome (PMS), menstrual cramps, menopause (benefits with St. John's wort), vaginal dryness, mild depression (melancholy), hot flashes, night sweats, sleep disturbance. Fruits can be made into jams.
- BLACK HAW/VIBURNUM (roots, stems, bark): Antispasmodic. Menstrual cramps, muscle cramps, intestinal cramps, uterine prolapse, morning sickness, asthma, lowers blood pressure. Fruits can be made into jams.
- CHASTE TREE/VITEX (fruit): Premenstrual syndrome (PMS), breast tenderness. *Chaste tree extracts restore progesterone levels. Roughly equivalent to Prozac for psychological and physical symptoms.
- CRANBERRY/VITAMIN C (fruit): Bladder infections (prevents harmful bacteria, E coli, from adhering to the cells that line bladder and urethra). *See herbal practitioners for kidney and bladder stones, incontinence, prostate problems.
- DONG QUAI (roots): Women's tonic, kidney tonic, menstrual cramps, PMS. Do not take with Coumadin or Warfarin.

CHINESE PRACTITIONERS... Circulatory, respiratory, reproductive, relieving headaches, infection inflammation, lowering blood pressure.

- RASPBERRY LEAF (leaves): Women's tonic. Pregnancy aid...

strengthen, tone, and relax. Smooths muscles of uterus and pelvis. Shortens labor, eases delivery. Regulates menstrual cycles and decreases heavy menstrual flow. Cleanses wounds and skin ulcers, as a gargle, and to stem diarrhea.

- SHATAVARI… Adaptogen (roots): Overall tonic for well-being, PMS, menstrual cramps, menopause, enhances fertility, breast milk production, indigestion, preventative for stomach ulcers, equal to Zantac.

WELLNESS AND PERCEPTION

- ASHWAGANDA… Adaptogen (roots): Anti-inflammatory, anti-anxiety, anti-arthritic. Rejuvenating tonic for strength and vigor, calming properties, boosts immune system, combats insomnia, aids anemia. Used for 4,000 years in India.
- BACOPA (above ground parts): Anti-anxiety, cognitive and memory, learning, helps focus, lengthens attention span, increases concentration. Used for 3,000 years in India.
- GINSENG PANAX… Adaptogen (roots): 500-1000 mg taken 1x or 2x daily. Overall tonic, reduces blood sugar levels in diabetics, immune system function, combats inflammation.
- GOJI BERRIES (fruits): Anti-inflammatory, antioxidant. Skin irritations, nosebleeds, joint pain, general well-being, lowers blood pressure. Avoid using during chemotherapy, radiation, or if taking Warfarin or Coumadin.
- GOTU KOLA (leaves and stems): Anti-inflammatory, antioxidant. Memory and cognition, circulatory problems, wound healing, fosters collagen.
- RHODIOLA (roots, rhizomes): Stress, anxiety, depression, fatigue, normalizes cortisol levels.
- SCHISANDRA… Adaptogen (berries, leaves): Treats diseases of: lung, liver, kidneys, heart, mental function, physical stamina, sexual performance, hepatitis. Do not take with high blood pressure or diabetes. Effects hypothalamus, pituitary and adrenal glands.

(An "adaptogen" is an herb that primarily increases the body's resistance to physical, biological, emotional, and environmental stressors. In other words, an adaptogen is traditionally thought to normalize or balance the body's energetic responses).

I hope this article gives you new insights into natural, simple healing that counteracts the use of drugs that are so-o-o-o prevalent in our world today. You will benefit tremendously if you study other sources on herbs. GOOD HEALTH is the single most important factor in your LIFE.

Here's to Herbs

Needing to plant dill for the pickle recipes I picked up at my farmers market, I pulled a book off my gardening bookshelf, *The Good Herb*, by Judith Benn Hurley. She has written articles and books on healing foods for the past thirty years and her information is right on target. I was surprised and impressed at the remedies she offered and believe you would be as delighted as I was to learn their uses.

- BASIL: Chew a sprig to freshen breath; essential oil treats skin conditions including acne, as well as sluggish, congested complexions. Basil also adds aroma to food and enlightens your mood.
- BAY LEAF: Brings tangy flavor to soups, stews, beans, etc.; adds strong enough flavor to make salt unnecessary in cooking legumes (cooking beans with salt makes their skin fly off); steaming your face calms stressed skin.
- BEE BALM: Native Americans used it to alleviate the symptoms of head colds and coughs; we use it in tea to help respiratory infections and nasal congestion. It contains tannins, which can help control oily skin. As an added benefit, it attracts bees to your garden.
- BURNET (salad burnet): Great in salads, tastes like cucumber; helps heal mouth ulcers; three tablespoons of burnet leaves and a sprig of mint in boiling water, stored in fridge and strained, makes a liquid that cools and restores your skin in summer.
- CALENDULA: Flower petals treat minor cuts and burns, contains essential oil compounds that soothe inflammation and help new tissue form; tasty and healthy in salads; the cream aids chapped or cracked winter hands and lips.

- CHAMOMILE: A stress antidote, tea soothes nerves and irritability, both in drinking it or using it as a facial rinse; good after the evening meal to soothe digestion; treats restlessness in children.
- WILD CHIVES: Onion benefits without tears; linked to reducing blood cholesterol levels, lowering blood pressure, and helping to prevent certain types of cancer (best eaten raw, not cooked).
- CORIANDER (cilantro): Ayurvedic herbalists claim it cools a hot stomach, banishes intestinal gas, and generally aids digestion; removes mercury from your brain.
- DILL: Dill seed tea relaxes and settles cranky stomachs; dill seed oil is an old-fashioned cure and preventative for chapped hands and split nails, also a large contributor of calcium to the diet, helping prevent loss of bone mass.
- ECHINACEA: Stimulates the immune system; treats infections; helps purify the lymphatic system; fights off colds and flu.
- FENNEL: Relieves intestinal gas; soothes symptoms of head colds; hot tea temporarily relieves respiratory congestion; helps nursing mothers produce milk.
- FEVERFEW: Soothes a headache; repels insects from culinary herbs such as basil in your garden (but keep away from plants that need pollination, such as fruits, since bees hate it and won't come near it when it is blooming).
- GARLIC: Raw garlic prevents and cures infection; helps lower blood pressure and blood sugar; helps prevent certain types of cancer by stimulating the immune system, increasing the body's ability to produce cancer-fighting interferon, and reducing the body's stress from pollution; contains germanium, a mineral that can help prevent cancer cells from reproducing.
- GINGER: An effective remedy for indigestion and nausea, heals motion sickness from planes, boats, cars, or trains; morning sickness (crystallized ginger can be chewed to avail one of this remedy); a ginger foot bath is soothing, and soaking in a ginger bath is said to relieve tension, as well as minor aches and pains, removing toxins from the body.
- HOT PEPPERS: Soothe the pain of arthritis by rubbing hot pepper salve on the skin; capsaicin (the smell and taste of hot peppers) stimulates the flow of saliva and related stomach juices,

used in small amounts in meals; are a digestive and circulation tonic. Five of the most common fresh hot peppers, or chilies, are Anaheim, Banana, Habañero (hottest pepper in the world), Jalapeno, Serrano. Wear gloves when handling hot peppers. Or to help remove the capsaicin from your fingers, rinse them in cider vinegar, rub with toothpaste, and rinse the toothpaste away with vinegar.

- LAVENDER: Essential oil of lavender possesses antiseptic and healing properties on cuts, burns, scratches, insect bites, and blemishes; it is also used to banish mild cases of anxiety and depression and create calm and tranquility; fresh or dried flowers added to facial toner or aftershave lotion can help regulate an oily complexion.
- LEMON BALM: A mind and body tune-up; is an anti-spasmodic, calming the gastrointestinal tract; has relaxation abilities and a calming effect on the heart, nerves, and rest of body; helps relieve high blood pressure.
- LEMONGRASS: A jet lag formula from essential oil with other supportive oils; combats depression and bad moods; lemongrass tea for colitis; lemongrass leaves steeped in black tea and splashed on face helps control oily skin.
- LEMON VERBENA: Tea relieves intestinal gas; the aroma of a dried leaf or two in your pocket rubbed from time to time will lift your spirits.
- MUSTARD SEEDS: High in magnesium, a mineral that can help regulate blood cholesterol levels and help regulate blood sugar levels in insulin-dependent diabetics; gives energy to people with chronic fatigue syndrome; helps regulate an irregular heartbeat; in a foot bath to relieve respiratory congestion.
- MUSTARD GREENS: Excellent source of beta carotene, the plant form of vitamin A; is associated with lowered risk for certain types of cancer; also, a source of vitamin C that helps fight infection and prevent heart disease (best for you eaten raw).
- NASTURTIUM: The leaves contain a natural antibiotic, effective against respiratory conditions, or used as a cold and flu cure; in a salad, offers a healthy and clear skin tone. Roll a nasturtium leaf around your index finger, hold it in place with your third finger, and massage your gums and teeth using small circular motions.

Your teeth will feel sparkling clean and smooth, and your gums will be gently tingly.

- OREGANO: Is a digestive aid, improves dyspepsia.
- PARSLEY: Is an herbal multivitamin. Four ounces of minced fresh parsley contains more beta carotene (vitamin A) than a large carrot, almost twice as much vitamin C as an orange, more calcium than a cup of milk, and twenty times as much iron as one serving of liver; is a diuretic; helps control high blood pressure; bladder tonic; prevents infections. Sweetens breath after eating onions or garlic. (Can actually stimulate menstruation, so women who are pregnant or suspect they might be pregnant should avoid eating it in large amounts).
- PEPPERMINT: Peppermint tea helps soothe the stomach lining and fend off nausea and vomiting; encourages digestion by stimulating the gallbladder and liver, especially after a fatty meal; relieves flu symptoms; stops hiccups.Relieve itchy, chafed, or sunburned skin with a splash of tea. Other mints are: corsican, pineapple, spearmint, apple, curly, and orange.
- ROSEMARY: Tea is an antidote for stress; relieves headaches; for shiny hair as a rinse to combat dull buildup; in skin oil for a massage to calm. Prior to racing each day, Tour de France bicyclists drink tea with rosemary as a stimulant.
- TANSY: As a foot bath to soothe tired feet; in your garden to attract ladybugs and repel ants and aphids.
- TARRAGON: Raw in salad, helps regulate high blood pressure and strokes (contains high amount of potassium).
- THYME: Has antiseptic and antibacterial properties effective in keeping mouth and gums healthy; respiratory healing; with olive oil as a massage for neck, upper body, and feet. Helps rid the body of coughs, sore throats, colds, and cranky digestion.
- YARROW: Tea fights high fevers; is an external skin splash to tighten pores and firm the skin.

Amazing, isn't it, that the herbs we can grow easily in our gardens can give us so much health and pleasure. I live in an area with scads of deer, who eat almost everything we plant, but they do not eat herbs.

As an adjunct for those of you who want to deter the deer from eating your flowers and plants, here is a recipe I have used for the seven years I've lived in the Hill Country. Seven deer roam through my twelve acres three times a day:

SORRY, DEER... RECIPE

1 egg
1/2 cup milk
1 tablespoon Cascade dish soap
1 tablespoon vegetable oil

Add to one gallon of water, spray plants once a week or after a rain.

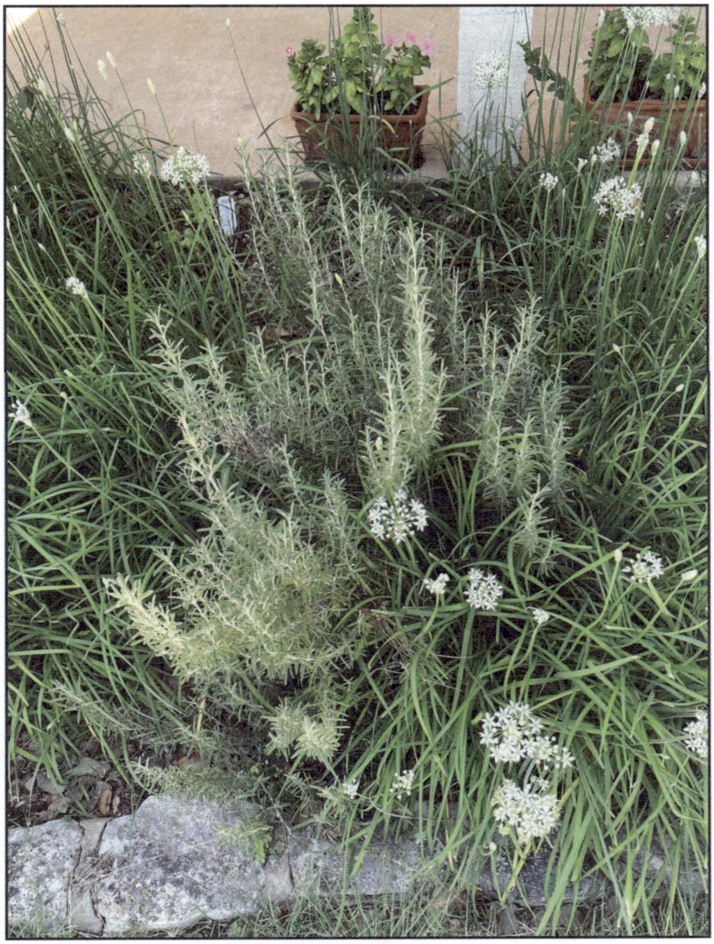

Fats and Cholesterol

"Good cholesterol is like a garbage truck
that goes through your arteries and
cleans out all the debris.
Cholesterol is a vital substance to the body.
Without it, we lose our memory,
weaken our immune system,
compromise our hormone levels, and
increase our chances of suffering from cancer."

(From *The Hidden Truth About
Cholesterol-lowering Drugs*,
by Shane Ellison, M.SC.)

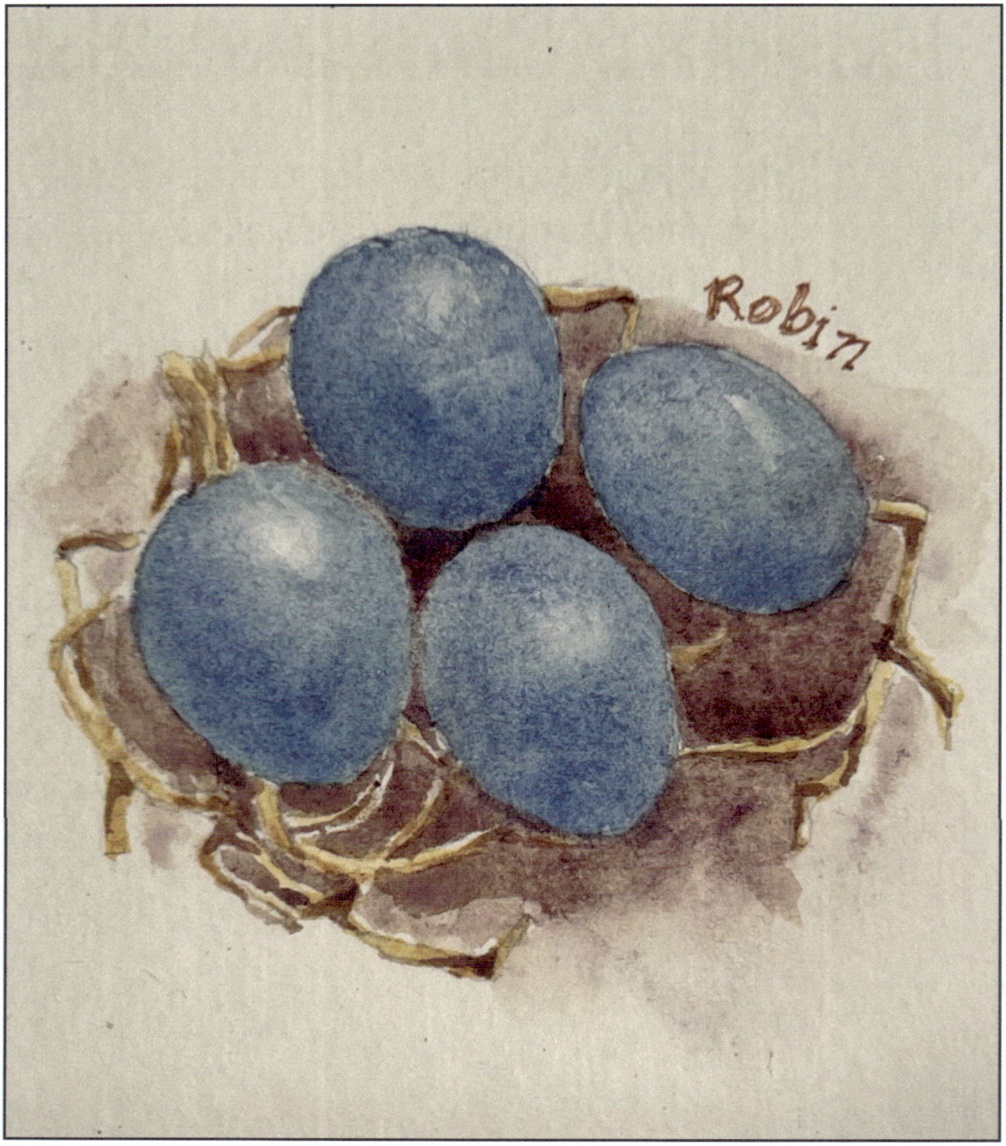
Robin

Dr. Weston Price

After nine years of deep and intensive research with alternative, cutting-edge doctors of nutrition and natural healing, I learned how important and necessary fats and oils are to a healthy human existence... the right fats and oils. And I learned how they have been maligned by food processors through advertising duplicity.

I became heir to major nutritional books from a researcher friend of mine, and received one I had been wanting, *Nourishing Traditions*, by Sally Fallon. Until I read her book, I had never known how important butter is.

In the 1930's, Dr. Weston A Price, a dentist here in the U.S.A., searched all over the world for peoples who were in prime health, had rounded faces and healthy mouths with no pinched, misaligned teeth. The tribe or village he found enjoyed superb health. They were free of chronic disease, were strong, sturdy and attractive; and they produced healthy children with ease, generation after generation. He brought back the knowledge of the foods they ate.

Thus, the Weston A. Price non-profit organization was born. In the 1980's, Sally Fallon championed it and brought this organization back into being.

Butterfat from healthy cows and goats has antimicrobial properties; that is, it protects us from viruses, yeasts, and pathogenic bacteria in the gut. They are directly absorbed for quick energy. They are less likely to add weight gain than commercial vegetable oils. These short-chain fatty acids are saturated and contribute to the health of the immune system.

Dr. Weston Price said, "The demonized saturated fats—which Americans are trying to avoid—are not the cause of our modern diseases. In fact, they play many important roles in the body chemistry:

Saturated fatty acids constitute at least 50% of the cell membranes, giving them necessary stiffness and integrity so they can function properly. They play a vital role in the health of our bones. For calcium to be effectively incorporated into the skeletal structure, at least 50% of the dietary fats should be saturated. They lower lp(a), a substance in the blood that indicates proneness to heart disease. They protect the liver from alcohol and other toxins, such as Tylenol. They enhance the immune system."

Butter is America's best source of important nutrients: vitamins A, D, K, and E. In fact, vitamin A is more easily absorbed and utilized from butter than from other sources. These fat-soluble vitamins occur in large amounts only when the butter comes from cows eating green grass without pesticides or insecticides. This butter's life-giving qualities are especially beneficial for children and expectant mothers.

Dr. Price found this deep yellow butter was exceptionally high in all fat-soluble vitamins and called them "catalysts" or "activators." He said that without them we are not able to utilize the minerals we ingest, no matter how abundant they may be in our diets. He also believed the fat-soluble vitamins were necessary for absorption of the water-soluble vitamins. Vitamins A and D are essential for growth for healthy bones, for proper development of the brain and nervous system, and for normal sexual development.

Many studies have shown the importance of butterfat for reproduction. As butter consumption in America has declined, sterility rates and problems with sexual development have increased.

Trace minerals are incorporated into the fat globule membrane of butterfat, including manganese, zinc, chromium, and iodine. In mountainous areas far from the sea, iodine in butter protects against goiter. Butter is extremely rich in selenium, high in antioxidant properties, and believe it or not, contains more per gram than herring or wheat germ.

Eat as much good quality butter as you like. Cook or sauté with it, use it as a spread on bread or crackers, bake with it... with the happy assurance that it is wholesome, indeed, an essential food for you and your whole family.

Good Fat... Bad Fat

Since the end of World War II, we the public have been the audience for insidious marketing by corporate entities such as pharmaceutical and food processing companies for greedy monetary gain. We have been consistently told that "FAT" is bad for us! Especially, saturated fat.

The result has been major disease. We have repeatedly been warned to eat low-fat or no-fat products. Do you know that our major organs: brain, heart, liver, and kidneys consisting of 50%-75% fat, are all dependent upon fat to be healthy? It must be good fat: organic coconut oil, walnut oil, avocado oil, macadamia oil, almond oil, olive oil, and butter.

Yes, *butter*, which we are warned time and again not to eat! And if you buy only grass-fed beef, lamb, goat, and pasture-raised chickens, their fats are healthy for cooking or frying our food.

"GOOD" fats we ate for years were switched to "BAD" fat replacements after 1950. Trans-fats are vegetable oils that have been chemically treated, heated, and hydrogenated, and are toxic, harming all our internal organs by oxidating (rusting) them. Trans-fats also change the low-density cholesterol (LDL) needed by our body, into L(pa) low-density lipoprotein, turning it into plaque in the major arteries around our heart. Inexpensive oils: soybean, corn, canola, safflower, sunflower, and Crisco shortening have been altered. Margarine is one of the most harmful foods you can eat, the primary source of trans-fats in the American diet.

(Put an unwrapped stick of margarine on your driveway in our summer's 100-degree weather. It will not melt, and no bug, butterfly or animal will taste it.)

All these create more work for our liver, which clears toxins out of our bodies. This way food is cheaply made to add $$$ to the processing companies' coffers, without thought of the harm it does to our bodies and our health.

These trans-fats are in 80% - 90% of all our grocery store purchases. Although, if the amount of trans-fat in a food is less than 1 gram per serving, the FDA allows food companies to list the amount of trans-fat as "0 grams" on the Nutrition Facts panel.

If you eat four or five servings, you could exceed 2 grams of trans-fats. There is no safe consumption of this food. It takes nine months to exit the body. Add to that the toxic Genetically Modified plants (GMO) that our FDA is corporate-paid to allow into our food chain without labeling… currently; corn, soybeans, canola, beet-sugar, non-browning apples, some squash, papaya, and alfalfa.

Unless you buy at Farmer's Markets or buy organic produce and cook it yourself, you are one of the many families being harmed. Before World

War II, mothers stayed home and cooked. After the war, mothers went into the work force and thus, food processing came about. We bought boxes, cans, jars, and packages of food prepared by corporations. It was easier on a working mother to buy instant dinners, whether in boxes or from fast food places: Whataburger, Kentucky Fried Chicken, etc. (These fast-food places that deep-fry French fries and meats, use soybean or canola oil that has become rancid after the first frying, and is toxic.) That has continued into today's market... everyone is too busy to cook at home after working all day.

For years, our allopathic, conventional medical system has connected high cholesterol and high saturated fat. It is a completely false narrative. It has helped them to sell statins to lower your cholesterol, and thus make billions of $$$. It is low cholesterol that will kill you.

Saturated fat is critical for the brain. Dr. David Perlmutter, M.D., an integrated neurologist, and a fellow of the American College of Nutrition says that both cholesterol and saturated fats are vitally important for brain health. A Mayo Clinic study, published in the *New England Journal of Medicine*, found that those individuals consuming the most saturated fat experienced a whopping 35% reduction in the risk for developing dementia. Saturated fat is a fundamental building block for brain cells.

Dr. Perlmutter says, "It's certainly interesting to consider that one of the richest sources of saturated fat in nature is human breast milk."

"The importance of breastfeeding your baby, especially during his first few months, cannot be over-emphasized. Breast milk is perfectly designed for your baby's physical and mental development. Breast-fed babies tend to be more robust, more intelligent, and freer from allergies and other complaints, especially intestinal difficulties, than those on formula. In addition, colostrum produced by the mammary glands during the first few days of a baby's life helps guard him against colds, flu, polio, staph infections, and viruses. Make sure if you use formula, that it does not contain soybean oil"... *from Nourishing Traditions*, by Sally Fallon.

Dr. Weston A. Price was a dentist in the 1930's who traveled the world over to find population groups untouched by civilization living entirely on local foods. They enjoyed superb health, were free of chronic disease, dental decay, and mental illness. They were strong, sturdy, and attractive, and produced healthy children with ease.

He found that they ate liberally of seafood or other animal proteins and fats in the form of organ meats and dairy products; they valued animal fats as absolutely necessary to good health; they ate fats, meats, fruits, vegetables, legumes, nuts, seeds, and whole grains in their whole, unrefined state. All primitive diets contained some raw foods.

In the 1970s, Sally Fallon restarted he Weston Price Foundation and her book, *Nourishing Traditions*, will give you invaluable information.

Our advertising media is there to make profit for the corporations they represent. Do your own research and no longer listen to marketing jazz. You also might want to read Dr. Mary Enig's, *Eat Fat, Lose Fat*, to learn the basics of oils and fats.

Statins and Cholesterol... What You Need to Know

The medical profession constantly warns us that we must lower our cholesterol levels or succumb to heart attacks or strokes from arteriosclerosis. Statins are the drugs doctors prescribe to lower cholesterol (Lipitor, Mevacor, Zocor, Pravachol, Crestor, Baycol, Zetia, Advicor, Altoprev, Caduet, Lescol, Simcor, Vytorin). For the past thirty years, the pharmaceutical industry has been running medical schools by educating their doctors in using these drugs, and profiting by multi-billions of dollars.

In 2005, the revenue from statins alone was $27 billion! What the public is NOT aware of are the damages of the side effects caused by statins.

Dr. Russell Blaylock, a renowned neurosurgeon for twenty-six years, stated:

> "Statins should be outlawed! They are one of the most harmful drugs ever created and have no more benefit than taking an aspirin a day as far as heart attacks. It's a SCAM! Cholesterol is NOT the cause of arteriosclerosis. The number one cause is over-consumption of dietary Omega-6 fatty acids, and no one is telling the public. Food sources high in Omega-6-fatty acids are oils such as corn oil, soybean oil, safflower oil, sunflower oil, canola oil, cottonseed oil, and several other related hydrogenated oils. The very oils they are

telling everybody they should eat because they're heart-healthy, contribute significantly to atherosclerosis! They are the source of Lp(a), the oxidized cholesterol that is damaging.

"They oxidize very easily, and this leads to inflammation that damages the arterial wall, which is considered the major mechanism for formation of atherosclerotic plaques and eventual blockage of the vessel by blood clots. This has been shown in a number of experiments. The most abundant oxidized oil in the wall of atherosclerotic blood vessels is Omega-6-oil and NOT CHOLESTEROL!

"There are other choices for lowering plaque, not cholesterol. Your diet can radically alter your cholesterol: cut out trans-fats, Omega-6 fats, and chemicals; consume Omega-3 oils (wild fish, free range chickens and eggs, pasture-fed beef, lamb and goat, wild game, and organic dairy), pomegranate juice and walnuts (ellagic acid), and many spices such as turmeric, ginger, cinnamon, etc. These stop the oxidation of lipids in the vessel wall. Oxidation results in the plaque we see in the coronary arteries and blood vessels to the brain."

(In *Breakthrough*, a major book on natural health and healing by twelve cutting-edge doctors, Suzanne Somers interviewed Dr. Blaylock... well worth your time to read.)

A survey of 1,700 patients with hardening of the arteries, conducted years ago by the famous heart surgeon, Dr. Michael DeBakey, found no relationship between the level of cholesterol in the blood and the incidence of atherosclerosis.

Oxidation of LDL (low density lipoprotein/bad cholesterol) comes from the wrong kind of fat; Omega-6 hydrogenated fats or trans-fats, which cause cells to become stiff or plastic. Omega-3 fats, such as the fat from pasture-fed beef, lamb, goat, and chicken, and wild animals, such as deer, bison, elk, and turkey, keep cells permeable, allowing body fluids to flow freely in and out.

Dr. Peter Langsjoen, a noted cardiologist in Tyler, Texas, says, "Removing or reducing statin drugs from heart patients' protocol IMPROVES their chances of surviving."

Dr. Nicholas Perricone, renowned dermatologist, in *The Perricone Prescription* writes "Statins cause increasingly dry skin and destroy the body's nutrients like CoQ-10, which promotes circulation in the body."

Dr. Joseph Mercola, author of the very well recognized and read e-mail medical newsletter, writes, "You must take COQ-10 which is central to the process of energy production in your body's cells (the mitochondria)."

Dr. Jonathan Wright, director of Washington's Tahoma Clinic, with medical degrees from Harvard and the University of Michigan, states that Merck and Company holds two patents on combining natural COQ-10 with statins to prevent a lot of the statin side effects, but are not using the combination because doing so might admit liability of statin drugs in liver damage.

In England or Canada, it is illegal to prescribe a statin without prescribing COQ-10… it leads to heart failure.

Doctors who seek to reduce patients' cholesterol levels with statin drugs face a serious challenge: lack of compliance. Among people who start taking statins, as many as 40% stop doing so in less than a year. Cost may be one reason, but side effects are another, even though many physicians may dismiss their existence.

Scientists at the University of California, San Diego, investigated how doctors respond to patient reports of statin related side effects. The findings, published in *Drug Safety*, might surprise you. Rather than reporting adverse events to the FDA, many physicians deny the drugs could cause undesirable symptoms, seem not to care, tell patients they are imagining pain, mistakenly attribute symptoms to aging, and refuse to believe or simply ignore patients' complaints.

Statins are responsible for the breakdown of cell walls; because of that, they are suspected to be the potential cause of neuropathy, a condition that causes nerve pain and dysfunction, and myopathy, a muscle-wasting disease that is now rampant in middle-aged adults. Another result can be myositis, a rare medical condition characterized by inflammation, causing blockage of the kidneys.

Dr. Mercola's July (2010) newsletter states that 900 studies proved adverse side effects of statin drugs: increased cancer risk, anemia, pancreas and liver dysfunction, cataracts, and acidosis.

Pharmaceutical America has set the cholesterol mandatory levels so low, 180 or less, that half of all adults in America are unnecessarily on a statin drug. Dr. Mercola says that 330 or less is within bounds.

Low cholesterol can lead to a host of other frightening problems: dementia, memory loss, lack of sex drive… and affect the immune system. Statins inhibit cholesterol production, depleting testosterone, estrogen, and progesterone. Testosterone is essential for building bone, muscle, and the sex drive.

Dr. Duane Graveline, an astronaut and flight surgeon, lost his whole memory for a week and had to be hospitalized, just from one dose of statin. He's written a book, *Lipitor, Thief of Memory*.

Cholesterol

The medical profession, drug manufacturers, and the media have so frightened and browbeaten the public into believing cholesterol and fat are enemies to our body, that we are convinced they must be avoided at all costs. (This has brought them billions of dollars in revenue.). Repetition of this hype has handicapped health logic among some of the most respected health experts in the world.

On the contrary, cholesterol and fat are essential to life!

"Good cholesterol is like a garbage truck that goes through your arteries and cleans out all the debris. Cholesterol is a vital substance to the body. Without it, we lose our memory, weaken our immune system, compromise our hormone levels, and increase our chances of suffering from cancer." (From *The Hidden Truth About Cholesterol-lowering Drugs*, by Shane Ellison, M.SC.)

Dr. Diana Schwarzbein, M.D., and Larry McCormick, consultant for Wellness Support Network: "Cholesterol and fat are used by the body as building materials for constant replenishment. Eating cholesterol and fat do not cause heart disease and accelerated death. In fact, you must eat them to avoid heart disease.

Cholesterol is a *type of fat* that has many functions in the body. Cholesterol is an important structure in cell membranes, keeping the cell membrane permeable so that liquids can pass easily through the cell. The inside of the cell is also filled with various cholesterol-containing membranes that must be maintained so that the cell can function well.

When you deprive your body of cholesterol, an essential building material, membrane structure is altered. When membrane structure is altered, cell growth is disrupted. As a result, there is a potentially higher risk of cancer because cancer arises from abnormal cell division.

Cholesterol is essential for brain function and the stabilization of neurotransmitters. Mood problems such as depression, agitation, and irritability can occur when your body does not get sufficient cholesterol. Cholesterol also forms insulation around the nerves to keep electrical impulses moving. Without this insulation, there is a rise in the potential for diseases of the nervous system, such as multiple sclerosis.

The brain and the gut both need cholesterol to reproduce new neuronal cells. Cholesterol helps the liver produce bile acids, which are essential for digestion of fats and rid the body of waste.

Cholesterol is an essential part of the myelin sheath. The myelin sheath is similar to the coating on copper wire and ensures that the brain functions properly by aiding the passage of electrical impulses. Without the myelin sheath, it is difficult to focus, and we can lose memory."

Eating the right kind of fats makes the difference in the quality of your life… eat real butter, not margarine! Stay healthy and enjoy life.

The Truth about Fats and Oils

If you read this for the first time last May and have not stripped your pantry, refrigerator, and freezer of every bottle, package, can, and jar of processed food that contains any of these destructive oils, then this is your second chance to avoid the degenerative illnesses they have brought about: *heart disease, strokes, arthritis, diabetes, obesity, cancer, etc.*

All disease is brought about by inflammation, and these man-made oils are major promoters of inflammation. These 'engineered' oils have lined the pockets of the national food processors with billions of $$$ and brought America to its knees.

We all deserve a second chance. *This is your second chance!*

Three years ago, when I read Bruce Fife's, "The Coconut Oil Miracle," and Dr. Mary Enig's and Sally Fallon's "Eat Fat, Lose Fat," I was shocked into angry action by all the misleading information and the outright lies fed to us by the Industrial Food Processing and Pharmaceutical Industries... all for greedy "BIG BUSINESS" profits!

Then and there, I decided to educate the duped public through lectures and written articles. I have been in mixed media advertising and marketing for twenty-five years and know: we believe whatever we see in magazines and newspapers or hear on radio and TV. I know, I was one of the believers!

In the mid 1980's the American Soybean Association stirred the media into a frenzy, criticizing coconut oil as a saturated fat causing heart attacks, and advised that it be replaced with hydrogenated vegetable oil, one of the most health-damaging dietary oils in existence. Healthy tropical oils were replaced with very nasty, chemically-altered trans-fatty acids (Omega-6) oils. This was to bring profits to the soybean industry that they felt coconut oil was usurping. Polyunsaturated fats from vegetable sources such as soybean, corn, canola, sunflower, safflower, and cottonseed oils show increased cardiovascular risk.

When these oils are processed by chemically adding hydrogen to extend their shelf life, they produce solid trans-fatty acids (the most damaging fats of all) to turn vegetable oils into shortening and margarine. These have brought us immune dysfunction, heart disease, strokes, diabetes, arthritis, obesity, and cancer in massive numbers.

Trans-fats (hydrogenated and partially hydrogenated oils) present a genuine danger to health. They decrease insulin sensitivity by making cell membranes stiff and inflexible. They depress the immune system. Measures such as changing from these oils to medium-chain fatty acid coconut, palm and flaxseed oils; mono-unsaturated olive oil; Omega-3 pasture-fed beef, lamb, and goat, organic butter, free-pastured chicken fat, wild animal fats, and wild Pacific fish oils can drastically improve the elasticity of each cell membrane to allow for hydration and oxygen to flow in and out freely. Cells that are hydrated and oxygenated work optimally and reverse the aging process to create a smooth functioning, healthy body.

Contrary to what we have been told, the fat from healthy animals is good for you, not harmful. We have been led to believe that fat consumption must be minimized, but we need fat in our systems, just natural fat, not engineered. Coconut oil is the purest form of oil there is and is not harmful even if you fry with it. It enters the body as energy, instead of turning to fat storage, and it does not interfere with your cholesterol. It increases your immune system.

Problem cholesterol is in the sticky Lp(a) that comes from Omega-6 oils that are oxidized! STICKY Lp(a) is what causes plaque in your arteries.

It is imperative that the meat you purchase is pasture-fed or wild, not corn-fed! Corn is what makes their fat marbleized (Omega-6) and they are also fed growth hormones and antibiotics and sprayed with pesticides. Feedlot containment does not lead to healthy animals.

Chickens get their nutritional value from being pasture bred, because their diet needs bugs, worms, plants and sun, not "cage-free" or "free range" (which hides the fact that there are hundreds or thousands of chickens in a barn with a door to go outside into a small porch area with a roof. But they rarely do, because they were born and raised inside, and the grain and water are inside).

Eggs from pasture-bred chickens are healthy and the yolks are more yellow and contain 50% less cholesterol than those bred in a chicken house. Seafood must be wild, not farm-fed (select Pacific or Alaskan fish, because there is too much mercury from industrial run-off in the Atlantic). Farm-fed fish are in troughs and usually plied with antibiotics and pesticides.

Dr. Khalid Mahmud, oncologist, says, "Eat God-made foods, not man-made foods."

The medical profession scared us about fats, as in olive oil, coconut oil, and other Omega-3 fats such as egg yolks from pasture-fed chickens. Wild game, and wild Alaskan salmon, halibut, sardines, and anchovies have Omega-3 naturally. Supplementing with Omega-3 fish oil capsules is important also.

Dr. Nicholas V. Perricone, nationally prominent dermatologist: "Omega-6 usage has doubled since the 80's; Omega-3 has shrunk 50% since the mid-1980's. Omega-6 in excess promotes: Inflammation, Increased Water Retention, Elevated Blood Pressure, Heart Disease, Cancer, Asthma, Diabetes, Arthritis, Depression, and Weight Gain" (emphasis added).

Cristiana Paul, M.S., nutritionist to doctors, in *Breakthrough*, by Suzanne Somers says, "When animals eat grass, their fat is high in Omega-3 oils, and when they eat corn in feedlot containment, their fat is high in Omega-6 oils. Farm-fed fish are low in Omega-3 EPA/DHA, which is what wild fish contain.

Harvard School of Public Health (published in the *Public Library of Science Medicine Journal*): "119,000 people die each year and 760,000 are in hospitals due to lack of Omega-3's in their diets."

Dr. Russell Blaylock, neurosurgeon, and author of *Health and Nutrition Secrets That Can Save Your Life*: "The number one cause of arteriosclerosis lesions is over-consumption of dietary Omega-6 oils. The very oils they are telling everyone they should eat because they are heart healthy. Canola oil is a mixture of Omega-6 and Omega-3 but has been shown to promote cancer. The most abundant oil in the wall of atherosclerotic blood vessels is Omega-6 oil and NOT CHOLESTEROL!!!" (emphasis added).

Harvard University Department of Nutrition, Nov.15, 1999:

"Replacement of partially hydrogenated fat (Omega-6) in the U. S. diet would prevent 30,000 premature coronary deaths per year." Epidemiological evidence suggests the number is closer to 100,000 premature deaths annually.

Dr. Mary Enig: "Powdered milk and eggs are added to reduced fat, milk, yogurt, and other dairy products to give them body (and do not state this on their label). These are damaged cholesterol (oxidized... caused by heat and oxygen) that can injure arterial walls and lead to pathological plaque build-up in the arteries. Contrary to what we've heard, cholesterol is not the cause of heart disease, but a potent antioxidant against free radicals in the blood... a repair substance that actually helps heal arterial damage. It is naturally produced in the body and naturally present in the foods we eat. No research has ever shown that cholesterol in natural foods causes heart disease. We have been pawns of the food and pharmaceutical industries."

In *The Perricone Promise*, Dr. Perricone says, "If you want radiant, supple skin, don't go low fat or no fat! Fat is the most abundant substance in the body, next to water. Fat provides energy, the building blocks for cell membranes. "

Polyunsaturated oils (vegetable oils) become toxic when they are oxidized as the result of exposure to oxygen, heat, or light (sunlight or artificial), causing rancidity and the formation of free radicals. Free radicals deplete our antioxidant reserves and cause chemical reactions that damage tissues and cells. By the time we buy oil in the store, it has already become rancid to some degree. These oils may sit around exposed to warm temperatures and light for months before they are sold. To make matters worse, the vegetable oils we buy sit in our kitchen cupboards for months. But, because pure vegetable oil does not produce any noticeable signs of rancidity, we assume them to be safe.

It is important to read the ingredients in any processed food, be it in bottles, bags, jars, cans, or boxes; and only purchase those with healthy ingredients. The major culprits are bakery products such as bread, rolls, cake, pie, cookies, crackers, muffin and cake mixes, mayo and salad dressings (even Crisco and Miracle Whip), soups, chips of all kinds, and breadcrumb mixes. To buy nutritious products, look for coconut or palm oil, olive oil, flaxseed oil, organic butter, avocado and walnut oils.

Your family's health depends on it!

Vitamin C… Wow… Surprise

Once in a while, we accidentally stumble across a hidden truth, one with such monumental implications that it staggers the mind.

I had planned on writing a column on vitamin C's importance to our immune system, and, as usual, picked up several books to research the subject: *Practicing Medicine Without a License*, by Owen Fonorow, *Why Animals Don't Get Heart Attacks… But People Do*, by Matthias Rath, M.D., *Vitamin C and the Common Cold*, by Linus Pauling, Ph.C., Ph.D., D.Sc., and *Stop America's #1 Killer*, by Thomas E. Levy, M.D., J.D.

I had no idea what a breakthrough I would come upon! In these books, I found a long suppressed medical discovery that could have saved millions of lives… and could have saved, fear, pain, and financial loss for untold numbers of Americans for the past twenty years – *if* the pharmaceutical and medical communities had accepted it in view of its efficacy.

Dr. Linus Pauling, one of our greatest scientists, the world's only two-time unshared Nobel Prize recipient (1954 and 1962), discovered our immense need for Vitamin C and wrote a book in 1970, *Vitamin C and the Common Cold*, about its importance in either preventing colds and flu or shortening their distressing symptoms.

In 1990 Dr. Matthias Rath, a German cardiologist, joined him, and they announced the co-discovery that cardiovascular disease is *caused* by a chronic vitamin C deficiency, not high cholesterol!

Vitamin C stimulates production of the collagen molecule; the most abundant protein built in our bodies and is *required* to keep arteries strong. Collagen stabilizes the walls of arteries to prevent deposits of plaque that cause heart attacks and strokes by narrowing the arteries, restricting blood flow, and causing angina pain. Collagen is laced through every cell, artery, vein, organ, bone, and muscle.

Their program recommends high Vitamin C to build artery strength, 3,000 mg. to 18,000 mg. daily (Vitamin C or ascorbic acid, has no lethal dosage).

With a Vitamin C deficiency, Lp(a), a sticky oxidized form of LDL, adheres to weakened arteries, causing plaque. Vitamin C deficiency can be corrected with major amounts of Vitamin C, and then the next step is taken. Two amino acids, L-Lysine and L-Proline, bind with Lp(a) to pull it loose and dissolve plaques, allowing the natural reversal of cardiovascular disease without angioplasty, stents, or by-pass surgery. This is the Pauling/Rath Vitamin C-Unified Theory and comprises the world's first health patented program to halt and actually reverse existing coronary artery deposits! Only a vitamin-based nutrient program provides the means for this healing process. Their program recommends high L-Lysine, 2,000 mg. to 5,000 mg. daily (L-lysine has no lethal dosage.)

Dr. Rath says, "Cardiovascular disease is primarily caused by chronic deficiencies of vitamins and other essential nutrients."

Dr. Rath and his team proved arteriosclerotic deposits can be prevented and even eliminated in the course of one year!

This world-startling news from Drs. Pauling and Rath in 1990 that there is no need for angioplasty, stents, or by-pass surgery, has been hidden not only from the public, but also from cardiac doctors and surgeons.

Why Has This Not Come To Light In Twenty Years? My blood ran cold with what I read.

In Owen Fonorow's *Practicing Medicine Without a License*, he states, "In over 50 years, not one medical pharmaceutical or government institution has done any scientific research on Linus Pauling's Vitamin C Theory!"

Neither the American Medical Association nor any medical journal has spoken of this because 'Big Pharma' runs the medical schools and decides what will be taught! The leading textbook for cardiologists, *Heart Disease—A Textbook for Cardiovascular Medicine*, does not mention Vitamin C one single time in 2,000 pages of teaching material for future cardiologists, despite the fact that the lack of this vitamin is the single most important cause of cardiovascular disease! It is a matter of record that the major medical journal, *Proceedings of the National Academy of Sciences*, refused to publish the Pauling/Rath "Vitamin C Unified Theory."

Mike Ciell, R.PH, of "our Health Co-op" wrote, "I find it practically criminal that, despite overwhelming scientific evidence, The Center for Study of Alternative and Complimentary Medicine of the National Institute of Health (NIH) has not done one clinical trial to test Pauling's and Rath's work. The Center is funded by tax dollars, so you would think that an incredibly affordable solution to the number one cause of death in this country would get some attention."

Heart Disease is Our #1 Killer!
It Has Become An Epidemic!

700,000 die each year in the U.S. and 12 million die worldwide.

The medical profession, drug manufacturers, and the media have frightened and browbeaten the public into believing that cholesterol is our enemy in order to sell their statins and other pharmaceuticals which have brought them billions of dollars in revenue. Repetition of this hype has handicapped health logic among some of the most respected health experts in the world.

Pharmaceutical America has set the cholesterol mandatory level so low, 180 or less, that half of all adults in America are *unnecessarily* on a statin drug. Dr. Joseph Mercola says that 330 or less is within bounds. Low cholesterol can lead to a host of other frightening problems, such as dementia, memory loss, lack of sex drive, and depression.

Dr. Duane Graveline, an astronaut and flight surgeon, lost his entire memory for one week and had to be hospitalized, just from one dose of statin. He has written a book, *Lipitor, Thief of Memory*.

The statins doctors prescribe for high cholesterol are responsible for the breakdown of cell walls, the potential cause of neuropathy, nerve pain and dysfunction, myositis, blockage of the kidneys, myopathy, and muscle-wasting disease. Statins, beta-blockers, diuretics, and other drugs are prescribed to treat the symptoms, and in so doing, bring about side effects. Have you ever read the small print that warns you against these?

Owen Fonorow states, "The American public is not told that their cholesterol-lowering statin drugs elevate the destructive, sticky Lp(a) at the same time as they reduce ordinary cholesterol! Canadian authorities require this warning in all advertisements. The FDA does not require this warning. So, American doctors are ignorant of this adverse effect… and there are no drugs that lower the lipoprotein Lp(a)."

Dr. Peter H. Langsjoen, one of the top American cardiologists from Tyler, Texas, wrote, "We are now in a position to witness the unfolding of the greatest medical tragedy of all time – never before in history has the medical establishment knowingly created a life-threatening nutrient deficiency in millions of otherwise healthy people. The top selling statin cholesterol-lowering drugs such as Lipitor and Zocor interfere with the body's synthesis of CoQ10, a vitamin-like molecule that our muscles require, especially the heart muscle, in order to do work. The shocking fact is that statin drugs cause muscle damage that leads to heart failure. Depriving the heart of CoQ10 is like removing a spark plug from your engine – it just won't work."

Dr. Russell Blaylock, neurosurgeon, "The number one cause of arteriosclerotic lesions is over-consumption of dietary Omega-6 oils. The most abundant oil in the wall of arteriosclerotic blood vessels is Omega-6 oil and not cholesterol!"

Harvard University, Department of Nutrition, "replacement of partially hydrogenated fat (Omega-6 fats) in U. S. diets would prevent 30,000 coronary deaths per year."

It is Omega-6 oils, these 'engineered' hydrogenated fats, such as soybean, corn, canola, safflower, sunflower, and cottonseed oils, that are responsible for oxidizing LDL and changing it into the sticky Lp(a) that causes plaque, *not cholesterol*! These oils are in cereals, salad dressings and mayonnaise, margarines, spaghetti sauces, soups, chips, cakes, pies, rolls, breads, breadcrumbs, etc., etc., etc. Read the ingredients!

Cholesterol is a *necessary* body substance, not a harmful one, as is advertised for corporate, medicinal monetary advantage.

From *Protein Power*, by Drs. Michael R. and Mary Dan Eades, "Cholesterol is absolutely essential for good health; without it, you would die. In fact, a grave sign of serious illness is a falling cholesterol level."

Cardiologist Dr. Diana Schwarzbein said it best, "The body uses cholesterol for constant replenishment."

Although medical, pharmaceutical, and media marketing have misled and frightened us about eating fats and oils, eating the *right fat* is imperative; these include: medium-chain fatty acid coconut, palm, and flaxseed oils; mono-unsaturated olive oil; Omega-3 walnut and avocado oils, organic butter, raw dairy, free-range pasture-fed chicken and eggs, pasture-fed beef, lamb and goat, wild fish, and wild game fats.

Dr. Nicholas Perricone stated, "Fat is the most abundant substance in the body, next to water. Fat provides energy, building blocks for cell membranes. Every cell membrane is 30% fat. More than 70% of brain and nerve cells are made of fat, making them resilient and shock resistant. Both cholesterol and fat are essential for growth in babies and children."

Don't be frightened by marketing ploys. Do some research. Everything is not what it seems at face value. Think for yourself. I have a normal IQ. I am not a genius. If I can discover these facts and truths, so can you.

Diseases and Conditions

The best solution is to prepare your own food
and to buy organic, non-GMO
REAL food products.
This not only avoids Alzheimer's,
but also heart attacks, strokes, and diabetes.

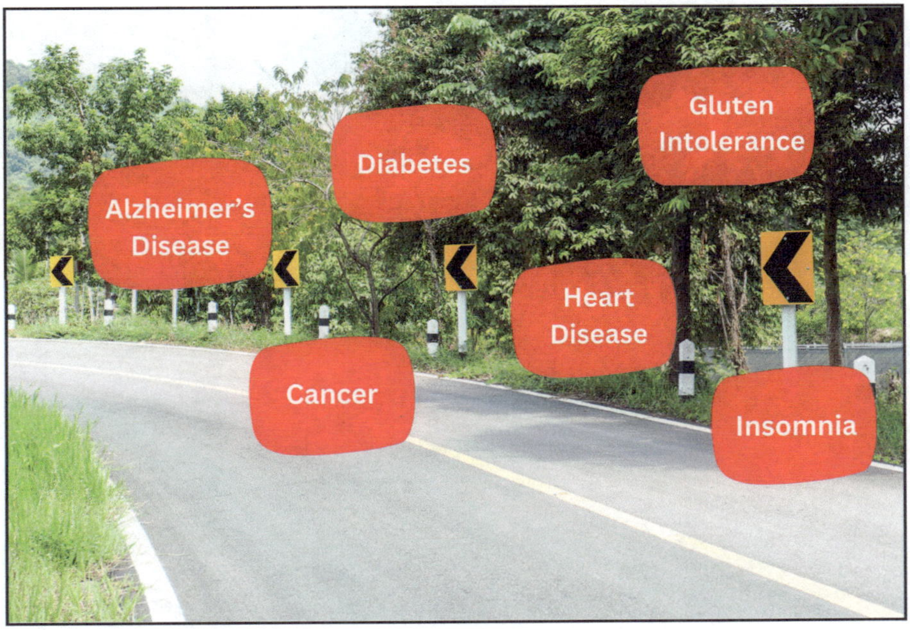

Alzheimer's

Alzheimer's is increasingly prominent in everyone's consciousness and frightens us because the number of people affected appears to be growing at an alarming rate.

It is not surprising that Alzheimer's is in the forefront of each of our thoughts, since the media notifies us of an enlarging number of Americans who fall prey to it each year, and orthodox medicine has been unable to make a difference in this relentless disease. It is the sixth leading cause of death in the US.

Breakthrough alternative naturopathic medicine, however, using natural methods and cutting-edge science, offers preventative strategies and some methods of reversing this sad disease. Early detection is an important start. *Nutritional deficiencies* are at the top of the list. The food we consume is responsible for building us up or taking us down, for reversing and correcting imbalances.

First and foremost is a deficiency in Omega-3 fatty acids and fish oil... vitamin A. Most processed foods in the grocery store and in restaurants contain the inexpensive Omega-6 trans fats: soybean, corn, canola, safflower, sunflower, and margarines (I Can't Believe It's Not Butter, Smart Balance) that oxidize (harm) all of our organs, including the brain. The secret to altering this is to read the backside of every package, can, and bottle you buy to be sure it is not infiltrated.

The best solution is to prepare your own food, and to buy organic, non-GMO REAL food products. This not only avoids Alzheimer's, but also heart attacks, strokes, and diabetes.

Don't tell me it costs more. Pharmaceutical drugs and medical appointments are way more expensive, and illness is not only costly, but miserable to live with.

The healthy oils are coconut oil, butter, walnut oil, avocado oil, olive oil. These build your immune system. Cook and bake with them and stay well. The chemical in fake butter is a catalyst for Alzheimer's. (Dr Jonathan Wright)

MSG and glutamates, chemicals purposely inserted into foods to tempt your taste buds and addict you, are called excitotoxins, because when brain neurons are exposed to these substances they become very "excited" and fire their impulses very rapidly until they reach a state of extreme exhaustion. Several hours later, these neurons suddenly die. (Doritos have three glutamates in their tasty chips).

The food processors hide them with other names: caseinate, protein isolate, autolyzed yeast extract, beef or chicken broth, natural flavoring and anything hydrogenated. It should be outlawed, but our FDA ignores the problem.

Doctor Roger Blaylock, a neurosurgeon for twenty-six years, said "Destruction of critical nerve cells in the temporal lobes plays an important role in Alzheimer's; consuming glutamates from childhood destroys these nerve cells. Consuming MSG and glutamates during our growth period produces grossly obese individuals. There is a strong link between obesity, metabolic syndrome, and Alzheimer's disease."

Detoxification of the human body is based on nutrition. The effectiveness of certain nutrients enhances the body's ability to detoxify environmental toxins. Fish oil and Omega-3 fatty acids stimulate brain repair. I use 10,000 iu of fish oil and krill oil, which comes from the smallest crustacean fish in the Arctic Ocean. The DHA in fish oil helps repair a lot of the damage that has been done, plus many B vitamins (thiamine, B6, niacinamide, B12, and folic acid) reduce inflammation, and inflammation underlies all disease.

Selenium repairs the immune system, so it repairs the brain as well. Deficiency of B12 also causes fatigue, hand and foot tingling, sleep disorder, and tendency to irrational anger. Soy depletes vitamin B12.

Pasteurization loses B12. Raw milk products retain all vitamins, minerals, amino acids, and enzymes that are also lost in pasteurization. Vitamin B12 is only found in animal protein. Vegans need an intramuscular injection once a month to defray anemia.

Anti-inflammatory nutrients, flavonoids, and carotenoids are a magic bullet. They shut down free radicals, produce anti-inflammation, and reverse the process of free radical generation. Flavonoids are plant pigments responsible for their color. Carotenoids are fat-soluble pigments.

NutraSweet and Equal, found in diet soda and other diet foods, are aspartames that cause brain lesions, aggravate and precipitate neurodegenerative diseases such as dementia and Alzheimer's, and cause dizziness and unbalance.

Massive deficiency of vitamins B1, B3, B12, folic acid, and zinc can cause dementia by allowing absorption of toxic metals such as aluminum. (Dr. Weston A. Price)

Aluminum, mercury, copper, and fluoride (fluoride is a sponge that permits aluminum into the body) are all heavy metals and toxic to the brain as well as to the entire body. Flu vaccinations also contain aluminum and mercury.

Chelation treatments remove heavy metals from the body and can sometimes reverse dementia and Alzheimer's. This is an intravenous process that removes blockage in arteries and veins and clears a lot of problems.

Fluoride, chlorine, and soybean products are iodine blockers. Iodine deficiency can be mistaken for Alzheimer's.

Vitamin deficiencies and overmedication are misdiagnosed as Alzheimer's 30% of the time. Sleep aids, tranquilizers, pain relievers, antihistamines, antidepressants, anti-reflux medications, antipsychotics, blood pressure medications, incontinence drugs, and anti-cholinergic drugs mimic Alzheimer's (Dr. Joseph Mercola).

A substantial number of Alzheimer's patients are victims of too many drugs or nutritional deficiencies that can be reversed. Estrogen disrupters from pesticides are found in patients with Alzheimer's. Also, poor and obstructed circulation may be a cause. The lion's mane mushroom stimulates growth of neurons and may play a role in inhibiting brain dysfunction. (Dr. Linda Page, "Healthy Healing")

The following foods and supplements are instrumental in preventing and healing, without chemical interference and without risking debilitating side effects:

Coconut oil and other medium-chain fatty acids increase the body's production of compounds called *ketones*. Ketones are compounds that are created when body fat is broken down for energy. Ketones are a powerful fuel for the brain, especially when the brain is injured or impaired. (Doctor Mary Newport cured her husband with three or four tablespoons of coconut oil in his daily oatmeal). Vitamin D3 and curcumin help digest plaque in Alzheimer's.

Omega-3 contains DHA, which is of particular importance for brain and eye health, and significantly improves cognition.

Wild blueberries guard against neurological diseases. Vitamin A and D3 are key antioxidants, beneficial for cell signaling and communication. (Dr. Fred Pescatore, New York)

People with the highest intake of vitamins C and E are least likely to develop Alzheimer's. (Dr. Linda Page) Lithium aspartate and lithium orotate block Alzheimer's pathways. (Dr. Jonathan Wright, Tahoma Washington Clinic)

All-natural protein melts away brain-clogging minerals that trigger memory loss, dementia, and Alzheimer's and cuts brain cell death in half (Nobel Prize winning discovery). 99% of doctors ignore this.

Eggs and butter are rich in vitamin A which feeds the hippocampus (the brain region breeding new cells) and are a key in the biochemistry of memory. (Dr. Pescatore)

These help halt progression of Alzheimer's: alpha lipoic acid, berberine, ashwagandha, astaxanthin, resveratrol, salmon, sardines, and anchovies.

Stimulating for the brain: puzzles, reading, and a business interest or goal.

I hope this article opens your eyes and decreases your fear.

"We have almost forgotten that our natural state is one of balance, wholeness, and vitality." (Sally Fallon, the Weston Price Foundation)

Drugs never heal, they abate.

Gluten Intolerance... and What to Do If You Have It

Each year more and more people are becoming aware they are gluten intolerant. One of every 133 people in the U.S. are in this category. This is also called Celiac disease, an inherited auto-immune disorder. The body mistakenly reacts to gluten as if it were poison, but gluten is actually a protein found in wheat and other grains.

The immune system reacts with an inflammatory response by destroying part of the small intestine villi that absorbs vital nutrients. It can lead to serious illness.

To be gluten-free, one must avoid eating barley, rye, triticale, bulgur, farina, kamut, spelt, matzo meal, semolina, and durham (also called durum), as well as oats, unless labeled gluten-free. It is also necessary to avoid processed foods that contain hidden gluten. (Once again, read the ingredient labels.)

Avoid: beer, breads, candies, cakes, pies, cookies, crackers, croutons, cereals, pastas, gravies, salad dressings, sauces and soy sauce, soups, frozen French fries, self-basting poultry, processed luncheon meats—unless labeled gluten-free, or made with corn, rice, or soy.

Watch for medications or vitamins using gluten as binders, hydrolyzed vegetable protein, natural flavoring, starch, texturized vegetable protein, toothpaste, or play dough.

Symptoms can include bloating, gas, diarrhea, abdominal pain, ulcers, IBS (Irritable Bowel Syndrome), weight loss or gain, constant fatigue or weakness, headaches, bone pain, a chronic itchy rash, infertility, or hallucinations. Children can develop canker sores.

Long-term complications, such as malnutrition, lymphoma, osteoporosis, miscarriage, depression, neurological complications, iron deficiency anemia, kidney disease, or cancer, can ensue.

Children's complications can be failure to thrive, short stature, distended abdomen, dental enamel defects, and unusual behavior changes. A typical child sees eight pediatricians before getting an accurate diagnosis.

Allowed: amaranth, arrowroot, buckwheat, rice, soy, corn and cornmeal, hominy grits, polenta, pure corn tortillas, quinoa, tapioca; rice, soy, corn, potato, or bean flours; fresh meats, fish, and poultry (not breaded).

Many groceries sell gluten-free foods. You can find frozen food sections and grocery aisles that have large signs pointing out this specialty.

Gluten-free diets may have low levels of iron, calcium, magnesium, essential fatty acids, fiber, thiamin, riboflavin, niacin, folate, Vitamin D, Vitamin K, probiotics. Vitamins B6, B9, B12 taken daily reduces homocysteine levels (harmful amino acid associated with higher risk of heart disease or stroke) and protect intestines from damage.

It is a good idea to get a blood test for antigliadin antibodies and endomysium antibodies. Then, a celiac panel to confirm.

The only treatment is to follow a gluten-free diet. The small intestine heals, and you return to full health.

Sources:
Dr. Joseph Mercola, gluten free.com
Dr. Julian Whitaker, gluten free.com
www.celiac.com

Reversing Alzheimer's: Some Very Exciting News!

If you've ever known anyone with Alzheimer's disease, you know how heartbreaking it can be. Not only does it destroy a person's mental abilities and dignity, but it wipes out the person's very personality, leaving behind a mere shell of a human being. The body is there for you to see, but the person you know and love no longer exists.

Alzheimer's is a scary disease. It seems to come without warning and, worst of all, until now there's been no cure. Named after the German psychiatrist who discovered it, Alzheimer's is a progressive, degenerative disorder that attacks nerve cells in the brain and leads to a disruption of memory, thinking, and normal behavior. In Alzheimer's, waxy clumps or protein fragments, called beta-amyloid plaques, form around and inside nerve cells, breaking vital connections and leading to nerve destruction.

Over 5 million Americans now have Alzheimer's. Currently, 10% of Americans over age 65 and nearly half of those 85 or older have the disease (worldwide, 26.6 million).

Alzheimer's appears to be one of the diseases linked to our "civilized" lifestyle. In less developed areas of the world, such as Africa, the disease is practically non-existent, which leads one to suspect that exposure to environmental pollutants and the un-natural food products so prevalent in our diets today play a critical role in this and other modern diseases.

A new breed of integrated, anti-aging, alternative doctors look to new solutions, and new premises. They search outside the box, not using the old status quo of "just treating the symptoms" of the disease with pharmaceutical drugs, but are healing the natural way, going for *the cure*.

They have each found a new approach, a hope for healing Alzheimer's. Frank Shallenberger, MD, HMD, medical director of the Nevada Center for Complementary Medicine, describes a colleague, Dr. Mary, whose husband Steve, of thirty-six years, was just fading away. He was known for his quick wit and sharp mind, could do complicated math in his head, take apart computers and repair them, enjoyed landscaping and kayaking. When his memory started failing, he got lost while driving home, couldn't even remember how to use a spoon, or how to get water out of the refrigerator. He didn't recognize close relatives.

Mary came upon an experimental drug that brought improvement in *half* the people who took it. She found out that the main ingredient of the drug was medium-chain triglycerides (MCTs) derived from coconuts. She went to the health food store and bought some organic coconut oil. When she started giving it to him, she asked him to draw a clock from memory. After two weeks of treatment, she had him draw a clock, again and, then thirty-seven days later.

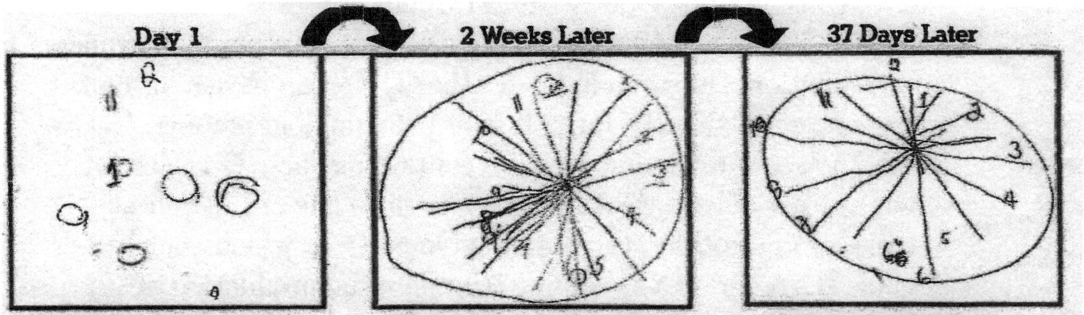

▲ This is what Steve drew when he was asked to draw a picture of a clock.

▲ This is what he drew after 2 weeks of treatment.

▲ This is what he drew 37 days later.

Just two months after he began taking coconut oil, Mary said he walked into the kitchen every morning alert and happy, talkative, making jokes. His gait was still a little weird, his tremor was no longer very noticeable, and he could concentrate on things, whereas before he was easily distracted.

Now, as time has elapsed, his gait is back to normal, and he jogs daily! His tremor is completely gone. He is once again an avid reader. He has also started doing volunteer work at the local hospital.

Dr. Shallenberger and Dr. Mary are convinced these changes are due to the coconut oil, because anytime Steve misses a dose, his Alzheimer's symptoms immediately return. He missed on two occasions and became dazed and confused, with full-blown tremors. In both instances he got back to normal after taking the coconut oil.

Dr. Shallenberger said when you add MCT oils to a low carb diet, the body is flooded with ketones, resulting in an amazing improvement in brain function. Ketones are a powerful fuel for the brain, especially when the brain is injured or impaired.

Both of these doctors' results are exciting and offer hope for the first time.

Following are steps you can take to protect yourself from Alzheimer's and memory loss. Natural foods and supplements are the key to protecting you:

- Blueberries have strong antioxidant capabilities, are a potent cancer preventative agent, help protect the heart and cardiovascular system, and are a potent agent against diabetes.
- Turmeric is one of the primary spices of Indian culture (average daily adult intake is estimated at 400 mg) and can lower the risk of Alzheimer's. India has one of the lowest rates of Alzheimer's in the world. Only 1% of its elderly suffer from it.
- Omega-3 fatty acids EPA and DHA are key components in proper brain function. Research indicates that DHA can have a dramatic effect on preventing the formation of beta-amyloid plaques. Eat foods such as salmon and sardines containing these Omega-3 fatty acids at least twice a week. Sardines are also one of the richest sources of nucleotides, the building blocks from which your body creates RNA and DNA, helping stimulate the production of neurotransmitters in the brain.
- One of the liver's primary roles is to detoxify the pesticides, pollutants, alcohol, and medications that produce a constant stream of harmful by-products. The liver transforms the amino acid lysine to create acetyl-L-carnitine. Acetyl-L-carnitine promotes better logical intelligence, verbal critical abilities, long term verbal memory, and selective attention. Acetyl-L-carnitine levels can be increased by eating lysine-rich foods: cottage cheese, dark meat chicken, fish, peanuts,
pumpkin and squash seeds, lima beans, lentils, and chickpeas. You can also take L-lysine supplements.
- Vitamins C, B3, B5, B6, iron, and essential unsaturated fatty acids also produce acetyl-L-carnitine.
- A natural extract from the seeds of the milk thistle plant, silymarin, triggers the regeneration of liver cells.
- Alpha lipoic acid stabilizes cognitive function with no side effects.
- L-tryptophan, an essential amino acid, facilitates the transmission of nerve impulses in the brain and nervous system through the formation of neurotransmitters. It is available in supplement form.
- Resveratrol, an extract from grape skins and grapevines, breaks up and removes the plaques in the brain. It might very well benefit others with memory loss or dementia.
- Protect your brain from chemical assault by avoiding contact with, and inhalation of, pesticides, herbicides, and toxic chemicals.

Studies continue to link these household, farm, and commercial chemicals to diseases of the brain.

- Get mercury, lead, cadmium, nickel, arsenic, and aluminum out of your body. Chelators (chemical compounds that bond to a metal ion and form a stable complex that can then be harmlessly carried out of the body) include vitamin C, yellow dock root, chlorella, and cilantro. Cilantro effectively removes mercury, lead, and aluminum.
- Minimize your exposure to aluminum. Don't use aluminum cooking utensils.

  Switch from spray deodorant to aluminum-free roll-ons, sticks, or alternatives.

  Avoid antacids (Maalox, Rolaids, Di-gel, Mylanta, Riopan), diarrhea medicines, nighttime pain relievers, sleep aids, antihistamines, antidepressants, incontinence drugs, and narcotic pain relievers which contain aluminum.
- Statins have been found to impair brain function. Studies have shown that statins increase the incidence of memory loss, inability to concentrate, impaired judgment, confusion, disorientation, irrational thinking, and other signs of dementia and senility.
- Walking, swimming, and cycling, which are aerobic exercises, increase blood flow to the brain, resulting in improved learning, memory, and attention ability.
- Do not use synthetic sugar replacement, aspartame, or MSG (or other glutamates).

These are just a few of the simple natural solutions the NEW breed of doctors have brought to the forefront. I hope it excites you as much as it does me!

(Not originally published in *Living Naturally Firs*t. This article was found in unpublished files.)

Treating Diabetes the Natural Way

Since it is a New Year, and since one out of three Americans, adult or child, either has the deadly scourge diabetes or pre-diabetes (insulin resistance), it is a fitting time to enlighten you with the information that type 2 diabetes can be REVERSED… with natural methods, instead of our continuing to be held hostage, with major side effects, by the presently used patent medicine prescriptions.

I have been writing this column for two years, and I am hoping that by now, you are aware that there are many diseases you take for granted as *hopeless* are *curable*.

- Doctor Julian Whitaker in California, who has been writing newsletters with factual information for thirty years or more, wrote a special report, *Dr. Whitaker's 3-week Diabetes Miracle*.
- Thomas Smith from Colorado, who cured his own diabetes, wrote the epic, *Our Deadly Diabetes Deception*.
- Dr. Jonathan Wright in Washington, who is probably the most revered doctor of healing breakthroughs, wrote *Your Self-Help Tool for Treating and Preventing Type 2 Diabetes*, *The Do-It-Yourself Guide to Natural Medicine and Optimal Wellness*, and *Beat Diabetes with This Miracle Spice*.
- Dr. William Campbell Douglass II, who wrote in his newsletter, *The Diabetes Cure You've Never Heard Of*; and from the Health Science Institute's research team, *Diabetes Defeated: from Insulin Dependent to Non-Diabetic in 6 Weeks Flat*… all of these objectively differing from conventional pharmaceutical corporations' views of 'treating the symptoms (for life!)'.

There is a safe natural way to prevent, treat, and even reverse diabetes, but unless you do your own deep research, you will never know about it. Dr. Whitaker believes that in 90% of cases, it is both preventable and treatable.

How do you know if you're at risk for type 2 diabetes? These symptoms might be early warning signs that diabetes is on its way:

- Excess weight-obesity is the most well-known symptom and easiest to spot.
- Skin tags: tags of skin most frequently found on the neck, under the arms, and in the groin area.
- Shin spots: slow spreading, brownish red, sometimes yellow discolorations of the shins.
- Dupuytren's contracture: connective tissue under the skin of the hand begins to thicken and shorten. It may pull the fingers down towards the palm of the hand as the tissue tightens.

You should also be aware of some internal risk factor clues: high blood pressure, elevated cholesterol and triglyceride levels, and/or a family history of diabetes.

There are ways to prevent and even reverse diabetes with natural, not pharmaceutical means.

Benfotiamine, a derivative of Vitamin B1 (thiamine), is both water and oil soluble, absorbs better than regular thiamine, and your cells hold onto it five times longer. Japanese researchers patented it in 1962 by and have used it successfully in Europe for the past fifteen years for the prevention and relief of symptoms of neuropathy.

This could be an inexpensive solution for reducing leg amputations, kidney transplants, coronary by-pass surgeries, atherosclerotic heart disease, diabetic retinopathy, radiological and laboratory diagnostics, less drug usage, and less renal dialysis. Benfotiamine has only recently been introduced into the United States.

A research team led by Dr. Michael Brownlee published the results of their study. An enzyme called transketolase provides a way for the cells to use up the glucose metabolites that are responsible for most of the damage seen in diabetes. It safely directs excess glucose to the correct pathway, offsetting potential cellular damage.

Benfotiamine boosted the activity of transketolase by 300% to 400%. Many researchers suggest beginning with a lower daily dose and then raising the amount every two weeks until benefits are being realized. 200 to 300 mg. per day for the first two weeks, then raise the dose to 300 to 450 mg daily.

You may need to increase your dosage to 400 to 600 mg daily, depending on the severity of your condition. Once you reach the ideal level for you, this becomes your maintenance dose.

Source: www.benfotiamine.net.

Jon Barron of Health Science Institute looked for botanicals that could help control blood sugar levels and help rebuild the organs that control those levels. He settled on four botanicals, two from the Ayurvedic tradition—fenugreek and gymnema sylvestre, the third from Japan—konjac mannan, and the fourth –the nopal cactus (prickly pear cactus) from Mexico. He calls it Glucotor.

There have been no clinical trials as yet, but one physician in Evansville, Indiana, Dr. Anthony Hall, tested it in his family practice on diabetics, and it produced results the doctors have not seen before, even with hard core drugs, including dramatic changes in blood sugar levels.

Source: www.baselinenutritionals.com

(This article was originally written in 2012. Baseline Nutritionals Co. is currently closed.)

Another possible combination of ingredients that may help blood sugar levels are a mushroom called *Afaricus blazei* that boosts adiponectin, a substance in our bodies that promotes normal blood sugar levels by helping your body use insulin efficiently, and a cucumber-shaped gourd in India called *Cocconia cordifolia*.

These steps are the simple way to reverse diabetes:

WATCH YOUR DIET.

Indigenous diets of fresh fruits, vegetables, and legumes have been replaced with processed, refined foods stripped of their natural fibers and nutrients. Fast food restaurants are a main source of eating out and are a major source of gaining weight.

Eat a low glycemic diet of fruits and vegetables. Buy organic so you get the nutrients missing in conventional groceries. Farmers' markets produce healthy produce, and you pass up the pesticides, herbicides, and insecticides in regular gardening.

Eat meat from pasture-fed animals. Their meat and fat are Omega-3, to counteract all of the Omega-6 hydrogenated fats in almost all processed foods (soybean oil, corn oil, safflower oil, sunflower oil, cottonseed oil, and canola oil are trans-fats, chemically changed and hydrogenated… Omega-6). You do need fats… use coconut oil, palm oil, olive oil, and organic butter.

Avoid starches… bread, muffins, cake, pasta, pretzels, chips, and sugar. STOP DRINKING SODAS! HIGH FRUCTOSE CORN SYRUP is the major cause of the obesity and diabetes epidemic. It is 600X as sweet as sugar.

Stop consuming artificial sugars: aspartame, Equal, Splenda, etc. They can actually make you gain weight and are very harmful to your body. Healthy sweetening can be had with natural sugars, Stevia, or Xylitol. Xylitol actually reduces dental cavity and plaque formation and builds bone. Dark chocolate with 70% cocoa is healthy.

Cinnamon aids your blood sugar levels... 1/4 tsp daily is a major aid in diabetes.

Two tablespoons of apple cider vinegar taken before a high carbohydrate meal works just as well as diabetes drugs, cutting the usual blood sugar surge in diabetics and those with insulin resistance and improving insulin sensitivity. Vinegar has no adverse effects and costs only $15-$20 a year.

Tea is one of the healthiest beverages on the planet. The caffeine and polyphenols in tea are thermogenic agents, meaning they help boost weight loss by revving up the rate at which your body burns fat. Chamomile and white tea appear to help lower blood sugar as well.

ESTABLISH AN EXERCISE ROUTINE.

Exercise helps normalize weight and controls blood sugar levels. Just a little weight loss does wonders. Aerobic exercise lowers blood sugar and burns calories. Resistance training, like weightlifting, builds muscle and improves long-term insulin sensitivity. Brisk walking is one of the easiest exercises, and a ten-minute walk after meals helps clear glucose out of the bloodstream.

The most important thing is to choose something and stick with it. Regular exercise resets your body's thermostat for hours after you stop exercising.

REPLACE VITAMINS AND MINERALS WITH SUPPLEMENTS FOR EXTRA SUPPORT.

Massive amounts of nutrients are lost as the kidneys rid the body of excess glucose by increasing urination.

Vitamin B complex (75 mg B6, 150 mcg B12, and 300 mcg Biotin) improves insulin sensitivity and helps prevent diabetic complications, particularly neuropathy.

Vitamin C (3000 mg), the most active antioxidant in our water-based tissues, lowers sorbitol, that sugar that collects in and damages cells of the eyes, kidneys, or nerves.

Magnesium (500-100 mg) because most diabetics tend to have low levels, and the lowest are most likely to have diabetic retinopathy and other eye problems.

Vanadium (100-150 mg) markedly lowers fasting glucose and improves other measures of diabetes. Vanadium is the most life-saving blood sugar supplement.

Chromium (200 mcg) helps insulin work better. It also has been demonstrated to facilitate weight loss.

Alpha Lipoic Acid (600-100 mg), which helps support peripheral nerve health and aids neuropathy, is both fat- and water-soluble, so it can enter all parts of the cell to neutralize free radicals.

Check out any of the doctors I mentioned at the beginning of this article; do your own research. The major author I suggest is Thomas Smith, who cured his own diabetes many years ago, and I believe you can do nothing better than to read his book, *Insulin: Our Silent Killer*. You might also want to read his 14-page manual that was in *Nexus Magazine* in 2004… "Our Deadly Diabetes Deception." It is the best information I have found, detailing the steps required to reverse Type II diabetes.

If you are taking drugs for diabetes or cholesterol, monitor your blood sugar and cholesterol levels to make sure they don't fall too low. Taper down your medications with caution. *Work with a physician!*

Since many conventional physicians may not be familiar with (or may resist) the idea of using even a well-researched natural product (in combination with diet, exercise, and other specific supplementation) while reducing or completely eliminating the need for a patent medication, you may want to consult one of the following groups for a referral to a skilled alternative physician in your area:

The American College for Advancement in Medicine, 800 532-3688, www.acam.org;

The American Academy of Environmental Medicine, 316 684-5500, www.aaem.com;

The American Association of Naturopathic Physicians, 202 237-8150, www.naturopathic.org.

Understanding Insomnia

Adequate sleep is essential for optimal health. If you are not alert and invigorated in the morning (like a multitude of others), require loads of coffee to wake up, and if you are dragging as the day goes on... you have not had enough sleep.

A lack of sleep affects everything: mental clarity, mood, physical energy, and immune function. Missing even one night of good sleep causes a noticeable decline in the activity of immune cells that fight infection. Sleep deprivation often results in sickness. Standard recommendation for colds or flu or other illnesses is "get a lot of rest."

Doctor Julian Whitaker of the Whitaker Clinic in California suggests a bedtime routine: go to bed and get up at the same time every day. Be sure your bedroom is dark. NO light. Even a small point of light disturbs the pineal gland at the back of your brain that harbors sleep. (The bedside clock is OK if the numbers are red, not white or blue).

The temperature of your room should be even. Avoid caffeine, alcohol, and strenuous exercise several hours before bedtime.

Wakefulness and sleep are governed by a 24-hour cycle, largely regulated by exposure to light and the secretion of hormones, particularly melatonin. As daylight fades, the pineal gland secretes melatonin, promoting sleep; your whole system prepares for sleep and your body processes slow down. Melatonin rises at dusk and peaks from 1:00 AM to 5:00 AM.

Evening showers help. Also, using a fabric bag of lavender under your pillowslip or lemon balm (*Melissa*) tea will naturally aid sleep. A magnesium capsule one-half hour before bedtime calms and soothes. Another little trick is to apply pressure between the big and the second toe for one minute.

Dr. David Williams, who for twenty-five years has written the medical newsletter "Alternatives," says you need to be exposed to bright light during the day to keep your internal day/night clock set properly. If you have to spend all day indoors, open the shades and curtains to let in sunlight.

What we need to do is treat the root cause of insomnia. Most insomnia is caused by body imbalances generated by some type of stress. It can be psychological or mental, physical stress like an injury, or precipitated by a medication. Once one of these stressors causes a troublesome period of sleep, your brain learns that new sleep pattern... and it's hard to break. Your body can actually train itself to not sleep. We need to fix the imbalance and retrain our body to sleep.

One major imbalance is cortisol. Stress causes your adrenal glands to increase production of the hormone cortisol, channeling extra energy to your muscles and boosting your blood supply to allow for quick action in a crisis. Energy is directed away from your digestion and growth process. If stress is chronic and continual, your adrenal glands become exhausted and instead of producing too much cortisol, they produce too little. Levels of cortisol rise thirty minutes before waking us in the morning, and then drop to the lowest point before midnight, allowing us to sleep.

With excess cortisol, you're hyper-awake, and your sleep is shallow, fragmented, and unrestful. If you are deficient in cortisol, you are awake at 2:00 AM and sleepy at 2:00 PM and feel tired all the time.

To treat deficient cortisol and rebuild your adrenal glands:

- stay away from processed foods containing refined sugar and flour, which are high glycemic carbs, causing your adrenal glands to work overtime.
- avoid more than one cup of coffee a day.
- take 500 milligrams of pantothenic acid (vitamin B5) two times a day. High stress depletes pantothenic acid.
- take 1500 milligrams of licorice herb two times a day, half in the morning and half at 2:00 PM. Cut down to 750 milligrams a day after one month. This helps by preventing your liver from breaking down cortisol.
- take adrenal complete extract 200 to 400 milligrams two times a day. I have found a source for all these remedies in one pill… call 1-800-791-3395. Ask for 'Adrenal Factor." The company is Advance Bio-Nutritional, and the cost is $34.95 per month.

Neurotransmitters, or the body's chemical messengers, cause the second imbalance. Four of the neurotransmitters are serotonin, dopamine, GABA, and endorphins.

Serotonin regulates mood, emotion, appetite, and the sleep/wake cycle. Deficiency is associated with insomnia, craving sweets and starches, being a night owl or perfectionist, depression, worry, anxiety, panic attacks, and obsessive thoughts. Drugs used to treat this are Prozac, Zoloft, and Paxil.

They can have serious side effects and interfere with other medications.

Natural alternatives are:

- 5HTP – 100 to 300 mg at 4 pm and again one-half hour before bedtime. It is effective in treating depression, fibromyalgia, binge eating associated with obesity, and chronic headaches, in addition to insomnia.
- Melatonin – 1 to 3 milligrams 1/2 hour before bedtime. Melatonin is stored in the pineal gland in the brain. As darkness comes, the pineal gland releases melatonin, helping you to fall asleep.
- Sex hormones (women) cause insomnia when low. Only bio-identical hormones work. Try progesterone cream first; you can buy it in any drug store or health store. Progesterone also builds bones. If this doesn't do the job for you, get a saliva test at your individual pharmacy. It will add the other sex hormones you need.

Dopamine helps regulate the sleep/wake cycle. A deficiency makes it hard to concentrate or focus, become easily distracted or bored, and may cause ADD or ADHD, apathetic depression (just don't care), or a craving for coffee. Drugs used to treat these are Ritalin and Adderall. They can be addictive and cause withdrawal symptoms as well as serious side effects. (Adderall recently was banned in Canada for increasing the risk of heart related deaths and strokes).

Natural alternatives are:

- reduce caffeine to 1 cup daily.
- take L-Tyrosine 1000 mg 3 times daily… morning, noon, and 3:00-4:00 pm.

GABA calms the body and slows down stress by blocking it. Deficiency symptoms are anxiety, panic attacks, seizures, becoming easily overwhelmed, finding it hard to relax, stiff or tense muscles. One of the drugs used to treat this is Valium. You can quickly become dependent, even in low doses.

Natural alternatives supplement with GABA's building blocks, amino acids that cross the blood/brain barrier and get to the brain where GABA is formed:

- Taurine - 250 milligrams 3 to 4 times daily. Helps increase GABA production, calms the body.
- Theanine - 100 to 200 milligrams 1/2 hour before bedtime. Reduces stimulating effects of caffeine and calms. A good remedy if plagued with thoughts of business, family, or money matters that you cannot turn off.

- Glycine - 500 to 1000 milligrams 3 to 4 times daily. Promotes deep sleep, no 'hangover' associated with sleep medications. Reduces daytime sleepiness and improves memory function.
- Niacinamide (the active version of niacin… vitamin B3) 1500 to 3000 milligrams 1/2 hour before bedtime. (Has the same results as Valium). Makes you calm and sleepy when the brain is going non-stop. Helps you fall asleep better, relax nerves, and even prevents diabetes. (Does not cause the niacin flush).
- Valerian root - 150 to 300 milligrams (standardized to contain 0.8% valerianic acid). Reduces tension, promotes sleep, especially if you suffer from both anxiety AND depression. Affords a more restful sleep.
- St. John's Wort - 200 to 400 milligrams daily. Works in two to three weeks. If you suffer from both anxiety and depression, take St. John's Wort and valerian root together.

Endorphins relieve pain and reduce anxiety. They produce feelings of euphoria and have a calming and sedative effect, with milder but similar effects as painkillers such as codeine, oxycontin, oxycodone, and morphine. These are highly addictive, especially to those who have endorphin deficiencies.

Natural alternative is:

The amino acid DLPA - 500 to 1000 milligrams 2 to 3 times daily. Works by preventing the breakdown of the brain's natural endorphins. Helps reduce pain, allowing for better sleep.

Warning: do not use DLPA if using monoamine oxidase inhibitor (MAO) antidepressants. This combination can create dangerously high blood pressure!

These therapies may work right away but can take three to six weeks to work. After six to nine months of these therapies, you can stop them, and you'll be sleeping on your own.

Publisher's note: No business relationship exists between the author and any products referenced in this article. The information is provided solely to aid those who may wish to use them in locating them.

Toxin Avoidance

Protect your brain from chemical assault by avoiding contact with and inhalation of pesticides, herbicides, and toxic chemicals. Studies continue to link these household, farm, and commercial chemicals to diseases of the brain

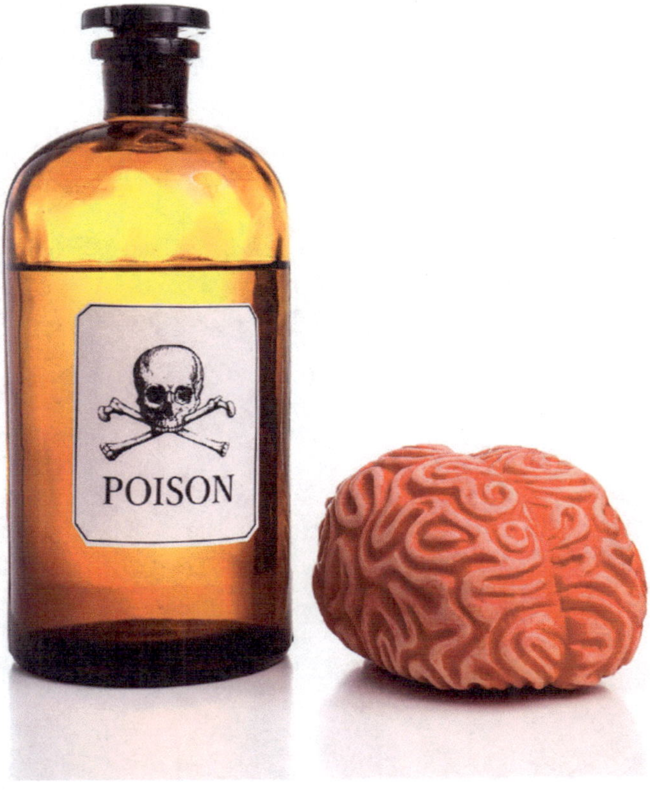

BPA—A Truly Harmful Chemical

Are you aware of how invasive plastic has become in our lives? And how harmful it is? BPA (Bisphenol-A) is a carbon-based synthetic compound that creates polycarbonate plastic, a clear, rigid, shatter-resistant plastic used to make a variety of common products.

These include baby and water bottles, sports equipment, medical and dental devices, dental fillings, sealants, CDs, DVDs, household electronics, eyeglass lenses, foundry castings, and water pipe linings. Along with epoxy resin, BPA was used in industrial solvents and high-performance coatings, *which line most of the 131 billion food and beverage cans made in the U.S. annually*. It was first synthesized in 1891 by a Russian chemist, A. P. Dianin; and it has been in commercial use since 1957.

BPA was formerly used as a fungicide. It infiltrates carbonless copy paper and thermal paper, which is most common in sales receipts. In this form, it is more readily available for exposure than when polymerized into resin or plastic. Handling thermal paper causes BPA to be transferred in the skin. The concern is over the residue on hands being ingested through incidental hand-to-mouth contact.

The European Union and Canada have banned BPA use in baby bottles. Canada declared BPA toxic. In 2010, the FDA identified possible hazards to fetuses, infants, and young children. Since that time, numerous studies have been performed at the National Center for Toxicological Research directed at many of those issues. Currently, the U.S. has no BPA labeling requirement for plastics. (*Editors note: Since the original publication of this article, the U.S. bans the use of BPA in baby bottles and children's spill-proof cups, also infant formula packaging materials.)

BPA's ability to mimic effects of natural estrogen enables it to trigger estrogenic pathways in the body. Exposure to BPA during pregnancy have caused possible health issues. And BPA has been found in high concentration in the placenta. Its hormone-like properties are exhibited, linking it to a wide variety of ills in fertility, breast and reproductive system cancer, and there is concern for neural and behavioral effects in infants and children.

Hyperactivity, attention deficit, and early puberty are also thought to be an outcome. Believe it or not, teething rings, plastic toys, books containing BPA that infants can chew on, have not been banned or recalled by the FDA or government agencies.

BPA may be linked to later physical and neurological difficulties. Concern about suitability in consumer products and food containers have had some retailers withdraw their polycarbonate products.

BPA is not an inert substance. I found the harm with which BPAs were charged included damaged chromosomes, reproductive problems, structural brain damage, increased fat formation, changes in gender-specific behavior, abnormal sex stimulation, diabetes, stimulation of prostate cancer, and alteration of immune function.

At least twenty years ago, my husband told me to get rid of all plastic food containers from my fridge, freezer, and pantry, and exchange them for glass. I buy raw milk that comes in plastic jugs, and I pour this milk into quart bottles. Buy bottles or waxed cardboard boxed food containers at the grocery store... no cans! (Higher concentrations of BPA have been found in canned beans, green beans, green peas, and chili.) Volunteers eating one can of soup daily for five days were found to have ten times the amount of BPA in their urine than when they ate freshly made soup.

Do not keep cases of bottled water in the trunk of your car or truck bed, because the heat increases the toxicity of the BPA in plastic bottles.

Do not microwave food in plastic containers.

Do not put plastics into the dishwasher.

Throw away, do not recycle, old plastic baby bottles, cups, dishes, and food containers with the letters "PC" for polycarbonate, or recycling label#7. The recycling will contaminate other products being recycled.

Do not recycle receipts or thermal paper as they will contaminate recycled paper.

When having a tooth filled or a root canal, ask if it is BPA-free.

Do not reach for the receipts for your purchases, let the seller put it in your bag. Please wash your hands after handling any receipt, so you do not touch your mouth, nose, or face without thinking.

Do buy Saran wrap and Ziploc bags that are labeled "product not formulated with BPA."

Now, you are aware of how pervasive plastic has become in our lives... and now you are also aware of how to counteract the problem.

Fluoride and Aluminum— Dangerous Body Toxins

"Fluoride is one of the most poisonous substances on earth," says Dr. Russell Blaylock, a brain surgeon for twenty-six years.

From *Webster's Dictionary*: "Fluoride-a compound of fluorine and one or more elements or radicals. Fluorine-a corrosive, poisonous, pale greenish-yellow gaseous chemical element, the most reactive nonmetallic element known, forming fluorides with almost all the known elements."

Yet, our dentists have been coating our children's teeth and telling us to use toothpastes and mouthwashes containing fluoride.

During World War II, we learned how to manufacture things from aluminum: airplanes, pots and pans, and buildings, to name a few. We also greatly increased our production of chemical fertilizers.

The downside of both these processes was a by-product called fluoride. Although it is a trace mineral naturally occurring in our food, in anything but those trace amounts, it's a more potent poison than arsenic.

Disposing of the thousands of pounds of fluoride by-products became a major problem in American manufacturing. They tried blowing it out their smokestacks, dumping it in our rivers, and burying it in the ground, but the immediate result was dead and deformed cows and other animals within miles of the smokestacks, rivers full of dead fish, and poisoned water aquifers. In fact, its primary use was as a rat poison.

Finally, the U.S. Public Health Service did a study that claimed to show that one part per million of fluoride in water reduced tooth decay by 60%, and thus began the trickling of fluoride into our water supply. The price of fluoride went up 1,000% almost overnight, and the problem of how to dispose of a potent toxin was solved.

Dr. Blaylock writes,

> "Fluoride is a waste product from the production of chemical fertilizer. We have to realize that it is a payoff system. Communities keep trying to refuse the companies selling it for the water supply, and they come back every year and try again. They offer the city contracts, government contracts, and dangle the possibility that they are going to do a big project if this community agrees to fluoridate the water supply.

"We now know without a shadow of a doubt that fluoride does not reduce cavities. It increases cavities. Even the ADA has been lying to dentists and the public all these years. Fluoride tends to accumulate, particularly in the bones, the thyroid gland, and in the brain. It lowers IQ. It's associated with Downs syndrome, and it triggers excitotoxity (destroying neurons in the brain).

"But the people who are promoting it, primarily the government and the ADA, have so much influence through the media that you really can't get the truth out. People are just not aware how enormously toxic fluoride is, particularly when combined with aluminum. Incredibly, aluminum is also added to drinking water to clarify the water. When you mix them together, which they do in drinking water, they combine chemically and form a substance that acts as a false transmitter for what is called G-protein receptors in brain cells, as well as other cells, and wreak all kinds of havoc.

"Tumors have these G-protein receptors and fluoride activates them. Fluoride increases cancer growth and cancer mortality. As you fluoridate the water, you fluoridate the plants. All over the United States we are seeing bioaccumulation of fluoride.

"There are only two ways to remove fluoride. One is a reverse osmosis filter. With reverse osmosis, the fluoride burns the filter, so it's important to replace filters nearly every three months. The other way to remove fluoride is to use a distiller, removing most of the contaminants.

"Most California wines have very high fluoride and aluminum levels. They use cryolite as a pesticide. Cryolite contains both aluminum and fluoride, which are very powerful neurotoxins. Cryolite is sprayed on the grapes, and it is then absorbed into the grapes.

"Once fluoride enters a food, it is impossible to remove. Fluoride is a very reactive substance, and it binds to the plant so you can't remove it. Sulfite in wine can produce significant excitotoxic damage. There is evidence that fluoride and aluminum, when combined, can greatly magnify the damage caused by the sulfite. Nearly all European countries have banned fluoride."

There are many problems with fluoride that we rarely hear about: Brenda Watson, R.N., President of Renew Life Formulas, says, "We were never meant to drink fluoridated water. Our digestive system is crucial and vital to our health and well-being, yet we put it to the extreme test every day by taxing its abilities to operate optimally."

Dr. Linda Page, noted naturopath, whose book, *Healthy Living*, has been published for twelve editions since 1985, states, "Watch your bottled water. Some brands contain fluoride. Fluoride toothpaste depletes Vitamin A. Also, causes allergies."

From the well-known Dr. Mercola newsletter, "Fluoride is in our cookware, microwave popcorn bags, stain-proof clothing, stain resistant carpet, flame retardants, food packaging from China, and household cleaners, toothpastes, and mouthwashes."

As for aluminum, it has crept into products we use every day. I was flabbergasted when I realized I had to ask for baking powder and for underarm deodorant *without* aluminum.

Aluminum is contained in night-time pain relievers, sleep aids, antihistamines, anti-depressants, incontinence drugs, and narcotic pain relievers.

Dr. Michael Galitzer, originally an emergency room doctor, and now practicing cutting-edge, antiaging energy medicine in Santa Monica, California says, "We've all stored our food in aluminum foil, are drinking soda in aluminum cans, cooking in aluminum pots, and are taking antacids containing aluminum: Maalox, Rolaids, Di-gel, Mylanta, and Riopan. These affect the neurological system. So, whether it's Parkinson's or dementia or slow thinking or forgetfulness, I look for heavy metal first."

Cutting edge, antiaging, naturopathic, homeopathic, alternative, and electric energy doctors (read *Breakthrough*, by Suzanne Somers) can detoxify your body with natural procedures.

Dr. Michael Murray, one of our most well-known naturopathic doctors says, "It impairs mental function and plays a role in Alzheimer's, Parkinson's, and ALS."

Dr. Blaylock stated that when we see the vaccination program with all its aluminum and mercury and over-vaccination effect, when we look at the food alteration and food additives, we're just going to see a lot more serious disease in younger people, and a severe drop-off in numbers of people who are able to reach their seventies and eighties.

He said that the *New England Journal of Medicine* published an article explaining that we're going to start seeing a decrease of Iife spans, because of exposure to environmental toxins.

The solution to all of this is to be aware of what you put in your mouth! Eat fresh food, not processed, not irradiated, not GMO. Read the ingredients with knowledge. Know that preservatives, additives, colorings, fake condiments, and chemicals are destructive to your health. The fewer ingredients on a label, the better.

These products are produced for their monetary advantage and to the detriment of your health. It is really easy to buy healthy food and achieve a happy quality of life.

Take back your power. Watch for errors like a hawk. Again, watch what you put in your mouth! THIS IS YOUR LIFE.

Genetically Modified Organisms: What You Need to Know

After World War II, there were a great many changes in our lives. Many of them were not to our betterment. Breadwinners had to work faster, longer, and harder to make a living; and the sacrifice was time. Life became more complicated. Both parents worked now, instead of only the father being the provider. The family was not as cohesive. New technology came into being: TV, computers, cell phones, DVD's, game-boys, Xbox, Wii, iPhones, iPads, and every other personal entertainment that separated family members from social togetherness.

A generation ago, not as many toxins were in our food supply. We mothers cooked three meals a day from fresh vegetables, meats, and fruits… with the whole family around the table, together.

Today, families generally pick up either a fast-food meal, frozen meal, meal in a box, a can, or a grocery quick-prep bag… each member eating on the run. The ingredients in these prepared foods are not always healthy. Unknown to most of us, for the past several generations many products have been introduced that have brought on illness.

One major product, Genetically Modified Organisms (GMO's), was created by five large corporations like Monsanto. GMOs are extremely toxic!

Genetically modified organisms are the result of laboratory processes that artificially insert *foreign genes* into the DNA of food crops or animals, which causes mutations. GMOs can be engineered with genes from bacteria, viruses, insects, animals, or even humans. A gene is taken out of bacteria to put into soy or corn seed, to make the plant immune to herbicides like Roundup and Atrazine. Then, thousands of acres of corn or soy can be sprayed, and only the weeds die. The *New York Times* reported that since Roundup has been introduced, there has been an 800% increase in myeloma of blood and bones (cancer). Atrazine is a suspected carcinogen and endocrine disruptor (thyroid, adrenal, and pituitary glands), and is a devastating threat to the environment. In fact, Europe banned Genetically Modified Organisms over twenty years ago.!

Jeffrey M. Smith, who is the internationally best-selling author of *Seeds of Deception* and *Genetic Roulette*, says there are two primary reasons why plants are engineered: to allow them to either *drink* poison or to *produce* poison. Poison drinkers are called *herbicide tolerant*. They survive otherwise deadly doses of toxic herbicide. The poison producers are called *Bt crops*. Inserted genes produce an insect-killing pesticide called Bt-toxin in every cell of the plant. When a bug attempts to eat the corn, its stomach splits open, and it dies right away. (Does that scare you like it does me?)

Dr. Mercola states on his Internet health newsletter, "The U.S. is completely unwilling to implement the precautionary principle with regards to *labeling* GM food, which is incomprehensible in the light of the findings we already have from animal studies."

So, it is very hard to know how to buy non-GMO foods. Right now, 70% of all processed foods, from baby food to chocolate, have GMO ingredients that are not labeled GMO. Every day you and I buy many name brands that we don't think about: Aunt Jemima, Quaker, and Argo corn meal or corn starch, canola and soybean oil in bakery breads and cakes, and salad dressings, to name a few. These foods look the same. They taste the same. The only way to purchase non-GMO is to look for certified 100% Organic or non-GMO labels.

In the produce section, look for the numbers on the stickers on the produce. You will find numbers, beginning with 9, 3, 4, or 8. The number 9 signifies it is Organic, the other numbers in the sequence signify it was raised non-organic or non-GMO. The number 8 signifies GMO!

In dairy products, if not labeled Organic, they may be injected with 'GM bovine growth hormone'. Look for labels stating "no rbGH, rbST, or Artificial Hormones."

GMO foods originated in 1996. The major genetically modified crops are: corn, soybeans, canola, sugar beets, cottonseed, Hawaiian papaya, and a small amount of zucchini and crookneck yellow squash. (Popcorn is not yet tampered with.) If sugar is listed as an ingredient, make sure it says, 'pure cane'; otherwise, it is mixed with GMO beet sugar. Avoid ingredients that contain corn sugar. This is from genetically modified corn (and is in fact high fructose corn syrup, with a name change, since the public has complained.)

Both Dr. Joseph Mercola, Jeffrey Smith, and the October 2010 *New York Times* have explained that Michael Taylor was first Monsanto's attorney, then recruited by the FDA (Food and Drug Administration) to head up the formation of GMO policy, then became Monsanto's vice president and chief lobbyist, and in 2009 was appointed as the *de facto* U.S. food safety czar at the FDA.

That is why the FDA denies knowledge of scientist's concerns and declares no safety studies on GMO's are required. The shocking truth behind GM foods and the huge effort by governments and big biotech corporations to keep information out of the mainstream media— and outside of your awareness—has been revealed in Jeffreys Smith's *Seeds of Deception*.

In fact, the American Academy of Environmental Medicine (AAEM) has publicly condemned genetically modified organisms in our food supply, saying they pose a "serious health risk." As a result, they called on the U.S. government to implement an immediate moratorium on all genetically modified foods and urged physicians to prescribe non-GMO diets for all patients.

The AAEM reveals a long list of disorders associated with GMOs. "Several animal studies indicate infertility, immune dysregulation, accelerated aging, dysregulation of genes associated with cholesterol synthesis, (faulty) insulin regulation, cell signaling, and protein formation, and changes in the liver, kidney, spleen, and gastrointestinal system."

From the *Indiana Business Journal*: "Proteins from GMO crops are showing up in Indiana waterways. Notre Dame and Loyola University looked at streams, drains, and ditches near cornfields, and found GMO bug-killing protein in 50 of them. When farmers mow the fields, residue remains from crushed plants, finding its way into waterways. GMO lingers. (Waterways were checked 6 months after harvest.)"

When Bt-toxin was sprayed over Vancouver and Washington State to fight gypsy moths, 500 people reported allergy or flu-like symptoms, and six went to emergency rooms.

In the *International Journal of Microbiology*, French researcher, Dr. Gilles-Eric Seralini of the University of Caen, concluded that rats that ate the GM maize had 'statistically significant' signs of liver and kidney damage. Female rats fed one of the strains also had higher blood sugar levels and elevated levels of fatty substances called triglycerides.

'Big Biotech' claims genetic engineering is a necessary step towards feeding the world's growing population, but GMO seed does not seem to be succeeding. India is a major producer of cotton, and GMO cottonseed has failed so badly that 150,000 Indian farmers have committed suicide in the past ten years because of crop failure.

All this information has been hidden by the FDA to keep the market from falling, but Monsanto's stock has fallen 42% since January.

Europe banned genetically modified food over nineteen years ago without government assistance, just educated consumers. And that was enough pressure on their food industries to drop their ploys. When consumers realize the dangers of GM foods and learn the FDA has abdicated its responsibility to protect us, they usually want to opt out of this massive feeding experiment. In fact, Most Americans already say they would avoid GMO brands, if given a choice.

But the FDA doesn't want to give us the choice. They ignore the wishes of nine out of ten Americans for mandatory GMO labeling to promote the economic interests of just five biotech companies. Genetically modified (GM) foods have *not* been scientifically tested on human beings.

The good news is that it wouldn't take a majority of us to kick GMOs out of our food supply. Kraft and other food companies wouldn't wait until half their market share is gone before telling their suppliers to switch to non-GM corn, soy, etc.

We can get them banned if we all band together and refuse to buy GMO foods. We only need 5% of our shoppers to stop buying foods with GMO ingredients. The millions in lost sales revenue would likely force brands to remove *all* GM ingredients, as they already have in Europe.

We already have these numbers on our side. 28 million Americans buy organic, 87 million think GMOs are seriously un-safe, and 159 million Americans, the majority, say they would avoid GMOs if labeled.

Let your grocer know that you will not buy GMO foods… then… USE YOUR WALLET TO MAKE YOUR OPINIONS KNOWN.

(Editor's note: This article was originally published in December 2010.)

Glutamates—The Brain Destroyers

The Truth Behind the Pervasive Food Additives

As a brain surgeon, and after twenty-six years of practicing neurosurgery in South Carolina, Dr. Russell Blaylock has recently chosen to devote his full attention to nutritional practice. He has authored three books on nutrition, one of which is *Excitotoxins: The Taste That Kills*.

He explains that excitotoxins are a special group of amino acids that are building blocks of proteins we call glutamate, aspartate, and cysteine. Food manufacturers add tons of these excitotoxic amino acids to foods of all kinds, including baby foods, because they greatly enhance the taste. MSG (monosodium glutamate) is a dangerous brain-toxic compound that should not be added to baby food or any other food. MSG is not the only taste-enhancing food additive chemical known to cause damage to the nervous system. A whole class of chemicals can produce very similar damage. They all share one important property. When brain neurons are exposed to these substances, they become very "excited" and spin themselves to exhaustion. Several hours later, these brain neurons suddenly die.

When people caught on to the danger of MSG, another substance called hydrolyzed vegetable protein was produced and is even more dangerous than MSG. Other names for these dangerous products are: caseinate, autolyzed yeast extract, beef or chicken broth, natural flavoring, soy protein concentrate, soy isolates, soy protein, vegetable protein extract. The government (FDA) has not made these illegal if they are not more than 99% pure. Some products say that there are no glutamates included, but the label lies.

The infant and child's brains are four times more sensitive to the damaging effects of glutamate than an adult's. It alters the developing child's brain, later causing abnormal menstrual periods, premature puberty, infertility, and learning and emotional difficulties. A favorite snack of children is 'Doritos'. Doritos have three glutamates in their chips and are 40% chemicals.

Hot dogs have a lot of MSG and are another favorite childhood food.

MSG in children causes grossly obese adults and adolescents. One small dose in children produces free radicals for two decades, causing chronic inflammation leading to arteriosclerosis.

Virtually every tissue in the body has glutamate receptors, and over-activation of these receptors can cause a wide variety of disorders including diabetes, heart failure, atherosclerosis, lung damage and can make cancers grow faster and spread throughout the body. In 1957, glutamates were found to be toxic to the retina of the eye… destroying it.

The obesity epidemic, the diabetes epidemic, the cancer epidemic, endocrine problems… all these things can be directly related to the intake of MSG. (Studies showed adding aspartame (Equal) to MSG greatly magnifies the toxicity and raises blood glutamate levels much higher than when either is used alone.) MSG has been shown to block the enzyme that has to do with the production of melatonin, so it can also produce insomnia. MSG scars the area of the hypothalamus that inhibits our ability to control appetite (removes the *trigger* that says, "I'm full.").

In 1945, after our soldiers came back from World War II, they found the Japanese rations tasted better than ours because MSG was added (produced in Japan). In 1970, our major food processors added 262,000 tons of MSG to American foods. Because we send food all over the world, we're seeing people from all parts of the globe having a problem with obesity, even in places where they never had it before.

Glutamates are in the great majority of our processed foods: breads, crackers, rolls, chips, bakery goods, cereals, salad dressings, spaghetti, soups, etc., etc., etc. The name of the game is SALES! What tastes good, sells. Food processors do not care what is toxic, they care what brings in the money. If we refuse to buy products with MSG and let them know, they will stop adding it.

The way to detoxify from excitotoxins like glutamates and MSG is to stop exposing yourself and your family. Read e.v.e.r.y ingredient on every box, bottle, jar, and bag of processed food! Then you do simple things that stimulate repair. Most important are things like DHA from fish oil. DHA is most beneficial for the brain and for everything else. DHA helps repair a lot of the damage that has been done… plus, a lot of B vitamins: thiamine, B6, niacinamide, B12, and folic acid. Also, selenium helps reduce inflammation, which is what leads to most disease. The foods providing powerful protection are flavonoids and carotenoids, naturally anti-inflammatory and antioxidant magic bullets:

- Flavonoid Plants—onions, letture, basil, garlic, cabbage, kale, Brussels sprouts, spinach, asparagus, fennel, lima and kidney beans, and garden peas
- Herbs—dill, tea, basil, thyme, cayenne, coriander, peppermint, chamomile, and anise
- Carotenoids—provide the bright red, orange, or yellow coloration of vegetables and fruits. They serve as antioxidants and are a good source of Vitamin A.

I don't know about you, but I can't afford to lose any brain neurons.

Hidden Dangers in Food Additives

If you have a party for children, or a football night for your friends, the first item on your table is a large bowl of chips as the prime snack food… to chomp on or dip in whatever sauce is in vogue at the time. It is the first choice of everyone coming to eat or nibble.

Are you aware that you are serving your guests some citric acid mixed with propylene glycol, a variety of glycerides, some propyl gallate, MSG, butylated hydroxy anisole, butylated hydroxytoluene, chemically altered fats, an excessive amount of sodium, GMOs, and of course, a measure of dyes and artificial flavoring? Still hungry?

When you buy a strawberry shake at a fast-food restaurant, do you know that the flavor is made up of forty to seventy chemicals from companies to create fragrances, like grape Jello?

Thirty years ago, in 1983, the FDA had approved the use of more than 3,000 food additives. Those listed as GRAS ("generally regarded as safe" at a specified level) totaled over 1,000. Today, some authorities estimate that as many as 9,000 chemicals appear in our foods.

The food industry spends *over 25 billion dollars* every year on the chemical additives included in our food. Americans eat approximately six to nine pounds annually. Your liver oversees detoxifying this garbage. As dangerous as one of these chemicals is in your body, a combination of several can be worse.

These additives are used mainly to make foods cosmetically attractive, to make them "convenient" to prepare, and to extend shelf life. These chemical additives serve a variety of purposes. They act as preservatives, drying agents, deodorizers, bleaching agents, curing agents, hydrogenators, antioxidants, defoamers, firming agents, etc. These are for *their* corporate profits, not for *our* benefit.

I imagine this partial run-down will surprise you:

BHA (butylated hydroxy anisole) and BHT (butylated hydroxytoluene) are used to prevent foods, in which the natural antioxidants have been refined out, from going rancid on the shelves over a long period. These petroleum-based chemicals have been banned in England and many other countries. You'll find them in cereals, candy, gelatin, shortening, ice cream, dairy foods, processed meats, peanut butter, margarine, chewing gum, vegetable oils, dried fruits, meats, fish, salad dressings and most popular snack foods.

LEAD – canned meats and milk may become contaminated with lead (from the seal on the can), but we unwittingly get it from toothpaste, aluminum foil, car exhausts, factory wastes, and various canned foods.

NITRATES pose an unnecessary cancer risk in combination with nitrosamines, found in cured and processed meats: ham, bacon, sausage, hot dogs, and cold cuts.

MSG or monosodium glutamate is an excitotoxin. Each time we eat a food with monosodium glutamate, it causes our neurons to dance in our brain, and some dance themselves to oblivion. (I need all the neurons I can get, don't you?) They have far-reaching results for other body functions, too. MSG makes food taste good and is addictive, so the food processors love it. It also removes the trigger that says, "you are full". So, you keep on eating and eating and eating.

GMOs are vegetables raised with seeds impregnated with the poisons of pesticide DNA and herbicide DNA. If a bug bites into one of these veggies, its stomach splits open and they die. These, too, have been banned in European countries.

ENRICHED BREADS contain *monostearates*, emulsifiers which cause flour to absorb up to six times its own weight in water. It acts on our tissues and cells. *Propionates* are used to slow down the growth of molds, making bread appear fresh longer. (Propionates are a prime ingredient in ointments and powders for treating athlete's foot.) They are steam-processed from ethylene and carbon monoxide and interfere with the body's ability to assimilate calcium.

Inorganic Calcium is the synthetic form of calcium used to "enrich" breads but cannot be assimilated by the body. *Ammonium Chloride* is used to ferment dough. You will also find this in antifreeze and powdered soaps and detergents. *Potassium Bromate* holds in air bubbles while the loaf is baking, providing a spongy texture.

Many home permanent products contain potassium bromate; the label carries a warning not to drink it. *Inorganic Iron* added to enrich most breads can't be used or assimilated by the body.

Chemically Altered Fats are in most breads. They are hydrogenated or partially hydrogenated and add Omega-6 oils to our bodies that are already supersaturated. They oxidize your organs and decrease your immune system. They are a major source of heart disease.

Refined Flour strips all the healthy fiber away and most vitamins and minerals are eliminated in the refining process. Fiber is a prime need in our diets.

SULFITES function as preservatives and/or antioxidants. Some are used as bleaching agents for food starches, some are used in the manufacturing of cellophane, and some are used as sterilizing agents. The only reason sulfites are added to our foods today is to improve the look of inferior foods and extend their shelf life. You'll find sulfites in baked goods, chip dips, fried fish, canned or dried fruits (especially in dried apricots), juices, gelatin, potato products, salad dressings, relishes, sauces, gravies, sauerkraut, coleslaw, shellfish (fresh, frozen, or canned), dried and canned soups, vegetables, (frozen, dried, or canned), vinegars, wine, beer, and cider.

ARTIFICIAL SWEETENERS are all addictive, and the health effects are profound:

*Saccharin (Sweet'N Low, Sugar Twin in the pink packet) has always had a warning on the package that it can cause cancer.

Aspartame (Equal and Nutrisweet in the blue packet) is a neurotoxin and penetrates the blood -brain barrier. Packaging contains a warning for dementia, Alzheimer's, Lou Gehrig's disease, and Parkinson's; and there is some controversy over it causing leukemia, lymphoma, and breast cancer.

*Splenda... when sales of Equal slowed down because it was causing headaches, this artificial sweetener was introduced. Open the yellow packet and pour it on the ants in your yard... they will be dead tomorrow.

Artificial sweeteners do not help you lose weight, they cause weight gain.

There are many other chemical food additives. The way to avoid them is to buy food at the farmer's markets, look for organic meat and vegetables, or raise your own. Eat *real* food, not processed in packages, boxes, bottles, jars, and bags. Cook your own meals like your mothers and grandmothers did. I raised four children, held down a full-time job, and still made all our meals, so don't tell me it can't be done. Maybe our lifestyle is faster now than it was in the 50's, 60's, 70's, 80's, and 90's... and maybe that is why we are sicker than we ever were in the past. If you don't have time to prepare your own meals, maybe it is time to slow down.

READ all the ingredients on a package. If you can't pronounce it, don't buy it.

If you stop buying the products with additives in them (products are on the market without additives), you will be voting with your pocketbook. Companies do not continue to produce a product that does not make a profit.

High Fructose Corn Syrup - The Truth Behind the Pervasive Food Additive

Dr. Jonathon Wright of the Tahoma Clinic in Washington State said that High Fructose Corn Syrup (HFCS) is the major cause of our epidemic proportions of obesity and diabetes.

The University of Colorado at Denver Health Sciences Center stated that the rising amount of fructose equals the increasing rise of obesity. One hundred years ago, the rate of obesity was only 5%. Obesity causes high blood pressure. Drinking 2½ cans of soda per day increases high blood pressure as much as 87%.

Dr. Chae Tracy, a Texas Hill Country chiropractor, wrote, "High Fructose Corn Syrup is a hidden source of sugar in a plethora of foods. Regular use is to blame for the skyrocketing rates of obesity and diabetes. European countries have banned its production due to health concerns. HFCS is big business in the U.S. and Canada. When consumers began questioning its use, manufacturers became up in arms. The Corn Refiners Association launched an aggressive marketing campaign, using television commercials and magazines, stating that High Fructose Corn Sugar is a 'natural' product and is healthy in moderation. It is not a 'natural' product, rather a science experiment gone awry with deadly consequences. The Food and Drug administration regulated the term 'natural', so there are many misleading labels on many foods. The beverage industry uses the most HFCS, followed by the processed food, bakery, cereal, and salad dressing industries. Always follow the money! First, it's cheaper to convert cornstarch into HFCS than to use cane or beet sugar. Second, it's easier to transport. Third, it has a longer shelf life."

The National Academy of Sciences' Institute of Medicine has found that diets with more than 25% of caloric intake from added sugars (excluding those of fruits and vegetables) significantly depress the essential nutrients… calcium, magnesium, and zinc.

Dr. Nicholas V. Perricone, *Seven Secrets to Beauty, Life, Longevity*, wrote, "High Fructose Corn Syrup was introduced in the 1970's. The 2004 issue of the *American Journal of Clinical Nutrition* reported consumption of HFCS increased 1000% between 1970 and 1990. HFCS is the only sweetener in soft drinks and is 40% of sweeteners added to food. Soft drinks used to be 6 ounces. Now they are 12 ounces, so more is imbibed. It promotes toxic glycation end products, degrades collagen in our skin, and promotes deep wrinkles, diabetes, obesity, atherosclerosis, and non-alcoholic fatty liver disease. High Fructose Corn Syrup bypasses natural mechanisms that prevent overeating and makes the body think it's still hungry."

Dr. Linus Pauling, the Nobel Prize winner for Vitamin C research breakthrough said, "Fructose is infinitely worse for the metabolism than sucrose (sugar)."

Ninety percent of corn is genetically modified, which introduces foreign proteins and may cause potential risks not yet understood. Seventy percent of American cornfields are treated with the herbicide Atrazine, a suspected carcinogen and endocrine disruptor (thyroid, adrenal, and pituitary glands) and is a devastating threat to the environment. The European Union has banned the use of Atrazine.

The other herbicide used in the huge GMO cornfields is RoundUp. Since RoundUp has been introduced, there has been an 800% increase in myeloma of blood and bones (cancer). Dr. Russell Blaylock, a neurosurgeon, states in

Suzanne Somers' book, *Breakthrough*, "Toxins from pesticides and herbicides, even in extremely small doses, are powerful neurotoxins and they suppress immunity. Some of these chemicals can produce autoimmunity, and they are also very powerful carcinogens."

According to Dr. Maoshing Ni, fructose is stored as fat in your body and is responsible for weight gain (30% of it around the belly). Soft drinks contain caffeine, phosphoric carbonation (which depletes calcium in bones), HFCS, artificial coloring and flavoring, and preservatives... nothing good, but all damaging. He goes on to say it causes tooth decay, nutritional depletion, type2 diabetes, and heart disease.

What you must do when you shop is read the ingredient list on every product you purchase, in order to keep HFCS out of your kitchen and your family. Check the products you already have in your pantry and refrigerator. You will be surprised how many of them Contain HFCS.

If HFCS was taken off the market, it would send the soft-drink industry into a tailspin, along with virtually every other food manufacturer!

(Originally published in June 2010)

Soy, The Misrepresented Food

All we've heard for the past six years or so is that to be healthy we must consume *soy* in all forms. It was written about and advertised in newspapers and magazines. Radio and television talk-show hosts expounded on it as a dietary need. We believed all the hype so sincerely that the stores latched on to the public response and filled every department with soy products. They certainly wouldn't miss sales!

The American Soybean Association must have been active again, as they were in the 1980's when they promoted a million-dollar media blitz condemning healthy coconut oil and opening the way for soybean oil and the other trans-fats and hydrogenated oils to enter our food chain. They have been a major cause of degenerative diseases in epidemic numbers for the past thirty years: heart attacks, strokes, cancer, obesity, diabetes, arthritis, etc. These illnesses came about a little at a time, so we became inured to them and did not realize how they have multiplied to an incredible degree. (You've heard the story of the frog who was put into a pot of cold water that was heated just a little at a time, until, when it became red hot, it was too late to jump out—he was boiled.)

Dr. Mary Enig, an international expert on fats, (the original researcher who discovered trans-fats) and Sally Fallon, CEO of the Weston A Price Foundation (the largest U. S. nonprofit foundation for food health and nutrition), wrote in *Eat Fat, Lose Fat: What's Wrong with Soy?*

"Today, many dieters try to meet their health requirements by eating foods based on soy, promoted as beneficial in many popular books and weight-loss plans. However, soybeans contain several natural toxins, and high temperature chemical processing adds many more. As early as 1972, a soy industry textbook (*Soybeans: Chemistry and Technology*) listed a number of well-documented toxic effects from soybeans, everything from endocrine disruption to undesirable changes in many organs.

The most serious problem with eating soy while you're trying to lose weight is that soy is a goitrogen, that is, it depresses thyroid function. When your thyroid gland malfunctions, you tend to gain weight even when you eat very little.

Dr. Dan Sheehan and Dr. Daniel Doerge, government researchers at the National Center for Toxicological Research, discovered the anti-thyroid component of soy is the isoflavones or phytoestrogens, which inhibit the syntheses of thyroid hormone. All soy foods, including tofu, soymilk, protein bars, and meal replacements, contain these thyroid-inhibiting isoflavones. In 1999, these researchers actually wrote a letter urging the FDA to require a health warning on soy foods, rather than the health claim the agency eventually approved.

(*Surprise, surprise, where have I heard that before?*)

What's more, the effects of soy food can be deceptive. Dieters who rely heavily on soy often report initial weight loss and energy increase, since at first the thyroid gland works harder to counteract the effects of soy isoflavones. But after a time, the thyroid gives out, with hypothyroidism the result. The dieter rapidly regains the lost weight, and then gains even more, plus, the dieter feels lethargic, unfocused, cold, and sometimes depressed.

And soy contains other anti-nutrients: phytic acid blocks mineral absorption, and enzyme inhibitors block the enzymes needed for protein digestion. Animal studies carried out in 1974 indicate that soy protein isolate, the major ingredient in modern soy foods, creates increased requirements for vitamins D, E, K, and B12, and deficiencies in many important minerals. Long-term consumption of high levels of soy foods can lead to serious nutritional deficiencies-definitely the wrong way to go if you are trying to lose weight.

Yet, the U.S. government allows a health claim for foods containing soy protein, and many government agencies and health organizations encourage consumption of large amounts of soy foods.

Promoters of soy for weight loss point to the Asian diet, which they claim contains a lot of soy. In fact, soy consumption is relatively low in Asia, ranging from an average of two tablespoons per day in Japan to two teaspoons per day in China. Even so, thyroid problems are widespread in Asia, particularly in China."

Linda Page, Ph.D., and naturopathic physician, in her 12th edition of *Healthy Living*, says a recent Hawaiian study suggests eating a lot of tofu may speed up the aging process, and even affect your brain.

She noted, according to the Maryland Nutritionists Association, soy may not be the best choice for infant formulas. Babies on soy-based formulas receive the equivalent of five to six birth control pills every day from soy's plant estrogen.

She also states soy foods are routinely genetically engineered (GMO), posing a problem for many people ethically and health-wise. People with food sensitivities are especially affected.

Soybean plants absorb manganese from the soil and concentrate it. Manganese is an essential nutrient, but in excess it is a potent neurotoxin. Baby formula may have 200 times the level that is in mother's breast milk. Such high concentrations can lead to brain damage in infants and altered behaviors in adolescents. Soy baby formula is easily considered one of the most dangerous food products on the market. These statements come from Dr. Joseph Mercola's web page.

Read Dr. Kaayla Daniel's *The Whole Soy Story*, where she says that unfermented soy has links to malnutrition, digestive distress, immune system breakdown, thyroid dysfunction, cognitive decline, reproductive disorders, infertility, severe and potentially fatal food allergies, danger during pregnancy and nursing, cancer, and heart disease.

Dr. Russell Blaylock, a brain surgeon for twenty-six years, blames soy protein, soy isolates, and soy protein concentrate as being harmful glutamates. In these, the glutamates (a natural amino acid) are too high, and it brings on a great number of maladies, including cancer.

According to Dr. Joseph Mercola's newsletter, from 1992 to 2006, soy food sales increased from $300 million to nearly $4 billion, practically overnight. This shift was no accident. It was the result of a massive investment in advertising by the soy industry that's been wildly successful.

Soy is indeed big business, very big business. From 2000 to 2007, U. S. food manufacturers introduced more than 2700 new soy-based foods.

As you can see from the following list, a large amount of scientific research shows that soy is not the nutritional panacea of the 21st century. Unlike the Asian cultures, where people eat small amounts of whole non-GMO soybean products, western food processors SEPARATE the soybean into two golden commodities: protein and oil.

And there is nothing natural or safe about these products. Soy contains hemagglutinin, a clot-promoting substance that causes your red blood cells to clump together. These clumped cells are unable to properly absorb and distribute oxygen to your tissues. Soy compounds mimic estrogen and may disrupt endocrine function. Drinking even two glasses of soymilk daily for one month provides enough of these compounds to alter your menstrual cycle. (Although the FDA regulates estrogen-containing products, no warnings exist on soy.)

So how *is* soy healthy?

Only one type of soy can be construed as a healthy food, and that is organic, fermented soy. Health-promoting soy foods include Natto, fermented soybeans with a sticky texture and strong, cheese-like flavor. It is very high in vitamin K2, which is a phenomenal vitamin, much like vitamin D. (Together, vitamin K2 and vitamin D provide a large number of significant health promotors, improving bone density and reducing your risk of heart disease and cancer.) Natto probably has the highest concentration of vitamin K2 of any food.

Tempeh, a fermented soybean cake with a firm texture and nutty, mushroom-like flavor is an excellent source of health-promoting natural probiotics. Miso, a fermented soybean paste with a salty, buttery texture commonly used in miso soup is also an excellent source of health promoting natural probiotics. Soy sauce, traditionally made by fermenting soybeans, salt, and enzymes, is another healthy choice. (Make sure it is a traditional soy sauce and not made artificially using a chemical process.)

Please note: TOFU is not on this list. TOFU is not fermented, so is not among the soy foods Dr. Mercola recommends.

Once again, you can live in health… just select the right products. It is smart to use your time and knowledge to live to a ripe old age with energy and enjoyment of life's pleasures. (Who wants to be a doddering ol' fool because you didn't pay attention early on?)

Sweeteners, Healthy or Toxic? We'll Let You Decide...

How many of us, while in a restaurant enjoying a delicious meal with friends, thoughtlessly reach into the little box of blue, yellow, or pink packets in the center of the table to sweeten our drink? I say 'thoughtlessly', because the majority of us are not aware of the toxins we are ingesting

Saccharin (Sweet'N Low, Sugar Twin, in the pink packet) was developed in 1957. It is made of petroleum and toluene, a solvent used to stop knocks in gasoline engines. We were later warned that it was linked to bladder cancer, but not many paid attention. Although saccharin is a chemical, the Mayo Clinic claimed it was a natural compound.

Aspartame (Equal, NutraSweet, in the blue packet) was developed by Searle Pharmaceutical Company and approved by the FDA in 1974. Aspartame is 200 times sweeter than sugar. There was so much controversy over its danger that it was held up until 1982.

Originally, three members of the FDA board turned it down, with only two accepting. Aspartame caused brain tumors in mice. But, Donald Rumsfeld, Secretary of Defense, who was a CEO of Searle, added two more board members and saw to it that it passed. It should never have been approved, but it was, over the objections of some of the major neuroscientists and toxicologists who served on the board of the FDA.

Dr. Russell Blaylock of Charleston, South Carolina, who has practiced neurosurgery for the past twenty-seven years says, "Aspartame breaks down into formaldehyde and formic acid and causes multiple breaks in the DNA associated with cancer induction. Studies show a dramatic increase in leukemia and lymphoma, also increasing breast cancer and probably brain cancer. It results in a tremendous increase in neurological diseases, particularly Parkinson's, Alzheimer's, and ALS (Lou Gehrig's disease). Aspartame is becoming a major addictive substance, and the health effects are absolutely profound. I find that a lot of women are drinking large amounts of diet colas, sometimes as much as a case in one day, because it's addicting."

Dr. Steve Nelson, founder and director of the Synergy Wellness Clinic in Palm Desert, California, said, "Diet soda, containing aspartame, is dangerous stuff, toxic and addictive, with cases reported of liver damage."

David Schmidt, inventor of LifeWave nanotechnology patches, states that we have artificial ingredients in our foods, two of which are Equal and MSG, both of which will create lesions in the hypothalamus. This is why people get a headache after having Chinese food. It's very simple; these artificial additives are giving us brain damage.

Aspartame penetrates the blood brain barrier and is a neurotoxin. Graves' disease is one of the results.

When sales of Equal slowed down because it was causing headaches, the manufacturers needed a new product, so Splenda (in the yellow packet) was introduced. Now most of the sugar- free food and drink products contain Splenda. Splenda is 400 to 800 times sweeter than sugar.

Dr. Steven Hotze of the Health and Wellness Center in Houston says, "Splenda is sucralose, which is a chlorinated hydrocarbon that is toxic. Any chlorinated hydrocarbon in the world is toxic, carcinogenic. Splenda was originally made as a pesticide... dump it on your ant beds and come back tomorrow to see all the dead ants. If you have to have sugar, just have a little sugar. It will be a lot better than eating poison."

Dr. Joseph Mercola, who is probably the most well-known Internet medical health newsletter writer, has written a book, *Sweet Deception*, all about the dangers of Splenda. He states liver toxicity is one of the side effects. Both Equal and Splenda will cause weight gain. They remove the little trigger in our brain that tells us that we are full. Instead, we keep eating.

The new information coming in is that fructose, or fruit sugar, can raise the uric acid level. (Gout is caused by too much uric acid.)

We have been told for years that fruit and fruit juice are healthy foods. Now, a number of sources debunk that.

Dr. Richard Johnson, chief of the division of kidney disease and hypertension at the University of Colorado, says that fructose promotes high blood pressure, diabetes, and obesity. Fruit juice is the culprit. (Fruit juice may be almost as hazardous to your health as colas.) Eating the whole fruit is better because you consume fiber along with the fructose. Little children of three or four, who carry extra weight and drink one or two sweet juice drinks a day, are at high risk, and double their risk of becoming seriously overweight one year later.

They should be given water instead of juice.

(Check the ingredients of the fruit juice you buy for High Fructose Corn Syrup content.)

Dr. Johnson has written a book, *The Sugar Fix*. You will find his Internet YouTube videos very worth your while.

Dr. Robert H. Lustig, professor of pediatric neuroendocrinology at the University of California at San Francisco's Center for Obesity, has also written a book, *Sugar: The Bitter Truth*. You can find his insights on the Internet, also. He writes that 50 to 100 years ago, we consumed 15 grams of fructose a day. Thirty years ago, it increased when high fructose syrup was introduced. Now, we eat or drink 75 grams a day, five times as much. Fructose is not metabolized like other food. It is converted into fat and stored.

Fiber in whole fruit contributes to a sense of fullness. Eating fiber also results in less carbohydrates being absorbed in the gut. Fiber consumption allows the brain to receive a safety signal sooner than it would otherwise, so we stop eating sooner.

Agave is a new high fructose sweetener, made from the agave plant. It has been mistakenly promoted for diabetics, but that is misinformation. Naturopath Linda Page, PhD. states in her twelfth edition of *Healthy Healing* that agave is 90% solids, a percentage much greater than traditional high fructose com syrup.

There are ways to satisfy your sweet tooth without the harmful effects of sugar:

Stevia is a natural green plant whose leaves have been used as a natural sweetener in South America for over 1500 years. It is non-caloric and about 25 times sweeter than sugar. One teaspoon of finely ground stevia powder equals one cup sugar in baking. It also is sold in packets for sweetening your drinks. It is a healthy alternative for diabetics and hypoglycemics and helps regulate blood sugar.

Stevia is effective for weight control because it contains no calories, yet significantly increases glucose tolerance. Research shows that stevia may block fat absorption, too. People whose weight loss problems stem from sugar cravings benefit most from stevia. When purchasing stevia, please read the ingredients, so you do not also get the other forms of sugar substitutes that processors can hide in there.

Xylitol is another sweet solution. It is made from either strawberries, plums, corncobs, or birch bark. It is safe for diabetics and hypoglycemics. Use in the same proportions as you would use sugar, whether in your tea or coffee, in baking, or for anything else you want to sweeten. It tastes exactly like sugar. Xylitol fights tooth decay (the opposite of sugar's cavity-producing quality), builds bone, and is now taking a role as an infection fighter with a nasal spray. Use it sparingly to begin with, because too much too soon may cause diarrhea for a short time.

If you insist on using sugar at times, buy turbinado, sucanat, raw, or evaporated palm sugar instead of white sugar, which has been refined with slaughterhouse animal bone ash as a filtering agent to remove the molasses, thus creating free-flowing white sugar.

Dr. Lustig says that food was just as abundant before obesity's ascendance. The problem is the increase in sugar consumption. Sugar both drives fat storage and makes the brain think it is hungry. Obesity is epidemic as a societal issue that pits the food-selling agenda of federal agencies and profit-seeking behavior of major corporations against public health needs.

Once again, it is monetary greed that drives them. The marketplace thrives on sales. If you don't buy food that is toxic, it will disappear from grocery shelves. It's your choice.

The Perils of Microwave Ovens

All of our lives are so busy today that we choose the easiest, fastest methods possible to live our lives, in order to achieve everything we have planned. We do not consider the cost to our health; we just continue and push through… but most of the time, we are not aware of what is unhealthy

Have you ever given thought to the harmful results your microwave causes, or do you only think of its importance and usefulness in doing the job in the short time you have to cook, thaw, or warm your food? We have used microwaves for decades now and take for granted that it is the easy way to cook.

"Heaven forbid" that we have to bake a potato in the oven for an hour, when it only takes four minutes in the microwave. How would we thaw our frozen meals? How would we melt butter? How would we reheat yesterday's dinner, quickly, for tonight? Why, every home we rent or buy always comes with an installed microwave oven! It is as expected as the sink in the kitchen.

There is extensive scientific literature concerning the hazardous effects of direct microwave radiation on living systems. It is astonishing to realize how little effort has been taken to replace this detrimental technique of microwave cooking with technology more in accordance with nature. Of all natural substances, the oxygen of water molecules reacts most sensitively. This is how microwave cooking heat is generated… friction from its violence to water molecules: structures of molecules are torn apart; molecules are forcefully deformed, and thus become impaired in quality. It is contrary to the conventional heating of food, where heat transfers convectionally from with-out to with-in.

Cooking with microwaves begins within the cells and molecules where water is present and where the energy is transformed into frictional heat. (Dr. Hans Hertel, Search for Health)

That same violent friction and de-formations that can occur in our bodies when we are subjected to radar or microwaves… happens to the molecules in the food cooked in a microwave oven. This radiation results in destruction and de-formation of molecules in food, and in the formation of new compounds (called radiolytic compounds) unknown to man or nature. (Tom Valentine, Search for Health)

Here is information from various informants, and they are many:

Sally Fallon, from Dr. Weston Price in *Nourishing Traditions*:

- Microwaves may have unfavorable effects on fats and proteins, making them more difficult to assimilate. Studies carried out in Switzerland revealed that the microwave caused changes in vitamin content and availability.
- Eating microwaved food results in abnormal blood profiles, similar to those that occur in the early stages of cancer.
- An especially dangerous practice is using the microwave for heating the baby's bottle. Altered amino acids in microwaved milk can be toxic to the liver and nervous system, especially for infants.
- Hamburgers cooking in the microwave tested muscularly weak; cooked in an iron frying pan resulted in strong muscle test results.
- Grocery store popcorn is rancid and is loaded with commercial salt and partially hydrogenated vegetable oils the harmful Omega-6 Trans-fats). Do not microwave in the aluminum metal container popcorn comes in. It exudes a harmful gas.
- Microwaves are powerful enough to rupture cell walls and alter protein molecules, causing free radicals.
- Enzymes are depleted. They are bio-active proteins responsible for virtually all of the major functions of the body. The first signs of

enzyme deficiency are indigestion, bloating, gas fatigue, and weight gain.
- After sixty seconds in the microwave, garlic's principal ingredient against cancer (Allinase) is rendered inactive.

Dr. Andrew Weil:
- Whole eggs cooked in the microwave have been known to explode on contact with cold air when the oven door is opened, and the scalding hot flying bits can cause nasty injuries.
- Boiling water in the microwave presents the same danger. It can splatter when you open the door.
- Don't heat food in plastic containers or covered by plastic wrap.

Dr. Lita Lee, Hawaii:
- Microwaved baby formula converts trans-amino acids into synthetic substances like trans-fatty acids. It converts one of the amino acids, l-proline, to a substance known to be poisonous to the nervous system and to the kidneys.

Japanese research:
- Vitamin B12, a vital nutrient, is another substance that can be destroyed by microwaving.

Dr. Hans Unrich Hertel, Swiss food scientist:
- Blood samples showed serious irregularities in the structure of microwaved food and in those eating microwaved food. These changes included a decrease in all hemoglobin and cholesterol values, especially the ration of HDL and LDL values.
- Lymphocytes (white blood cells) showed a more distinct short-term decrease following intake of microwaved foods than other cooking venues.

Dr. Joseph Mercola (prominent Internet spokesman):
- The convenience of the microwave becomes a significant toxic threat to you and your family. Microwaving causes a change in your food's chemical structure.
- Leakage of numerous toxic chemicals from packaging of common microwaved foods: pizza, chips, and popcorn. The chemicals included

are polyethylene terpthalate, benzene, toluene, and xylene.

- Microwaving fatty foods in plastic containers led to the release of Dioxins (carcinogens) and other toxins into our food. One of the worst contaminants, BPA (bisphenol A), an estrogen-like compound in plastic, reduces dishes that are specifically made for microwaving, and often contain BPA.
- Microwaving blood products before transfusion damages blood components.
- Don't stand near a microwave when it is running, especially if you are pregnant; definitely tell children not to stand nearby.
- Eyes are particularly susceptible to microwave radiation.
- A recent study showed unequivocal evidence that microwave frequency radiation affects heart rate and heart rate variability. It can cause blood sugar to spike and may be the cause of one type of diabetes (Dr. Magda Havas, Trent University.).
- Microwaves are used in the field of gene-altering technology to weaken cell membranes. Scientists use microwaves to actually break cells apart. Impaired cells then become easy prey for viruses, fungi, and other microorganisms.
- It is recommended that you resist using the microwave oven at all costs.
- The Jet Stream Oven uses convection currents and is a healthy alternative to the microwave. It does not compromise the taste of foods like the microwave and will even brown chicken and roasts.

Doesn't this information make you willing to take a little extra time and research in converting your cooking and heating methods in order to counteract all of the negative influences to keep your health intact?

I threw away my microwave oven several years ago, even though I work at two jobs, have a home to keep up, and am as busy as everyone else. It took some practice, but I cook, thaw, melt, and heat with ease, and with very little more time consumed in the process.

Knowing that electro-magnetic frequency is one of the most harmful products of modern-day technology, I am free of worry or fear about my body being subjugated to it.

Education allows us to learn methods by which to live, without the harm from modern discoveries.

I propose this as lesson #101.

(Editors note: This article was originally published in April 2015. Since that time, the public has become much more aware of BPA and other toxic substances about which the author warned.)

Memories and Recipes

Marna L'Amie was a force of nature–a one-of-a-kind woman. If one met her, that person would never forget her. Here are some thoughts from her children on what made her such a standout. Interestingly, several of the quotes are similar.

Bram Franklin –

I think of the lengths she went to protect her children. From marching into a school's principal's office to defend us, to checking out cupboards for toxic foods. She would do anything for her children. My other favorite thing was we didn't need permission to visit her. We just needed to tell her how many people were coming.

Reid Franklin–

A fierce, savvy protector of her children, while at the same time being patient and wise in raising her children.

Lynda Furgatch–

Mom was the epitome of hospitality: "You're welcome any time. Stay as long as you want." And, we loved her for her sense of humor and outrageous behavior.

Melanie Cox–

Mom loved hosting people. It didn't matter the color of your skin or your social status. She would be as welcoming to a garbage collector as she would be to the rich and famous. She never met a stranger.

Marna and I were such good friends and could talk for hours. We shared many memories of our long friendship back to the fall of 1951 when we first met in Coleman–my hometown. She and Jack had just arrived from Houston, and Frank and I had married in April of '51.

When we met that fall, she and I were two of a group of women who gathered to organize a bridge club. She was strikingly good-looking like a model, tall and thin with that black hair. Those were the days when we still wore white gloves most everywhere. It was a night meeting, and we all showed up wearing the proper attire, including white gloves. First, we organized the club, then had social time. Our hostess, Rita, served cake and coffee using her fine china and white linen napkins. All so fancy!

During the social time, Marna told about the time she and Jack had been in Mexico City and driven through the Redlight District. Well, in those days none of us ladies had ever discussed such a thing, and with that subject each one of us had dropped our head to concentrate on the cake and coffee. Looking back, I found it hilarious, as Marna and I laughed and laughed at the memory!

Later, at bridge club one day Marna began to talk about the hot topic, artificial insemination, the current article in the still-very-large-size *Life Magazine*. Again, everyone was so uncomfortable because we just did not have such discussions... I saw that Marna was sophisticated–from the city, and talked intellectually without inhibitions. To me, she was a "fresh breath" in town.

Letter from Frances (Burger) Stephenson

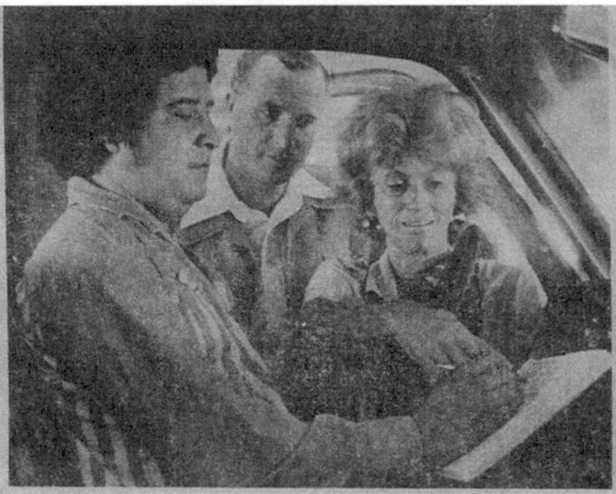

A new car

Joe Flores, from left, a make ready mechanic at Dan Hixson Chevrolet goes over a new car check list with David Bonds, Hamlin High School athletic director, who bought a new Hixson Chevrolet from Marna Franklin last week. (Staff photo by Jonny Cates)

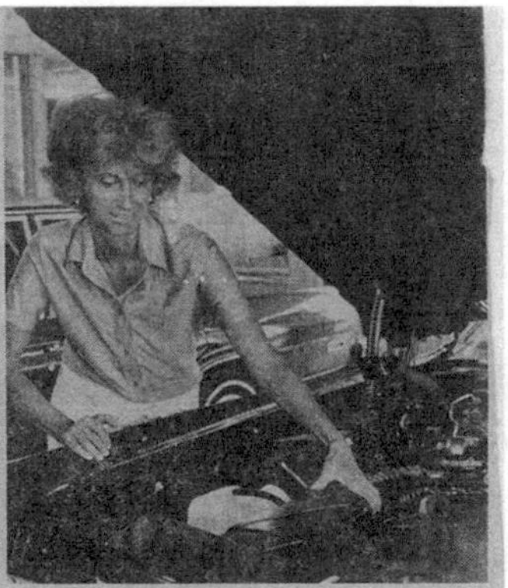

One of the boys

When Marna Franklin started to work at Dan Hixson Chevrolet, she knew the difference between a Ford and a Cadillac and that was about it. Now, she's just "one of the guys," she says. (Staff photo by Jonny Cates)

Air Intake Hose Is Elephant's Trunk

Car Saleswoman Redefines Engine Parts

By BEV MORGAN
Staff Writer

When you look under the hood of your car you'll see a hot water bottle made out of steel — that's a catalytic converter. And, you'll see something that looks like an elephant's trunk—that's an air intake hose.

This is how Marna Franklin, the tall, red-headed saleswoman at Dan Hixson Chevrolet, explains that confusing steel mass to her customers.

Men are very good humored about her simplistic approach. "I guess they just figure I'm a dumb female. . .so they laugh." Most women, on the other hand, appreciate her basic explanations.

When Mrs. Franklin first asked her husband, Jack, if he would mind if she applied for a job selling cars — he laughed, but told her to go ahead.

And a little while later, she told him, "They really like me, I think I'll get the job." He replied, "Oh, Marna, they're just humoring you."

But they weren't. In the spring of 1974, Mrs. Franklin accepted a job offer from Dan Hixson.

"When I first came here, I knew the difference between a Ford and a Cadillac and I knew you had to put gas in a car. That was about it," Mrs. Franklin laughed.

But after a week and a half of intensive training and hundreds of questions, Mrs. Franklin understood the "jumble" under the hood.

She remembered her first question. "I asked the salesmen, 'What's a carburetor.' " Their reaction was something close to hysterics," she said.

Mrs. Franklin said reaction to a female salesperson has been good in most cases. "I ran into one jealous wife though. She called me on the phone and said she'd look for cars for her husband by herself. . .for me to keep out of it."

Mrs. Franklin feels that women in car sales are valuable, because they relate better to women. Several women have told her, "It's so nice to talk to a woman about cars."

Women are more soft-spoken and they tend not to "hard-sell" a product, she added.

Working in a "man's world" has presented a few odd situations.

"I open doors for men (customers). The problem is, it's starting to get into my private life. I have to keep my hands behind my back to hold down the urge when I'm out in public," she laughed.

When she first came to work at Dan Hixson's she found the coffee pot was located in the anteroom of the men's restroom.

At first, she had someone get her coffee for her. But that took too much valuable time from her busy morning. "So I started yelling, 'every man for himself,' waited a minute and walked in."

Mrs. Franklin isn't just a saleswoman. She modeled for a few years and went to college until she got married. "I had four kids and stayed home with them. I really think you have to be with your kids when they're young," she said.

As her four children grew up, she went to college in computer science for a while. "I can understand astronaut talk now," she laughed.

Later, she went back into modeling. And now, she's working on a dual degree in art and business administration at a local college. "I'm gonna have those papers someday," she smiled.

When she first started work at Dan Hixson's, she said she felt "like I was diving into ice cold water and didn't know how to swim."

But, now, it's a comfortable and fun job, she said. "I meet hundreds of people and I love people."

"Of course," she laughed, "my mother always told me never to ride in a car with a stranger and now I take ten or 12 men for a ride a day."

There are two other women salespersons in Abilene. Cathey Rich who works at Toyota of Abilene and Isobel Shafer, who works at Cantrell Cadillac.

Kosher Dill Pickles

Ingredients:

25-30 Pickling cucumbers
4-6 Grape leaves
2 handfuls Fresh Dill
1 head Garlic, cloves each peeled and sliced in half
¾ box of Pickling Spice, cloves removed
Vinegar
Salt
Brine

For each gallon of water, add:
¾ cup salt, 1 cup vinegar

Place 2-3 grape leaves in bottom of large crock, clay pot, or non-reactive container. Place the cucumbers on top of the grape leaves, layering the stack of cukes with spices, dill, garlic, and placing remaining grape leaves in middle of the stack. Dissolve salt in water on stove.

Add vinegar and pour brine over cukes in crock until they just float. Adjust volume of brine for your container size. Cover cukes with plate (may need extra weight0 to hold them down and covered in brine.

*Half-dones will be ready in 7-10 days. Full done pickles will be done in about 12-14 days.

Marna's Marinated Salad

Ingredients:

2 green peppers sliced
1lb. mushrooms thickly sliced
½ cauliflower cut into bite size florets
1 cup chopped celery

Mix together:
1 cup oil
⅓ cup wine vinegar
1¼ tsp. salt
1 tsp sugar
½ tsp pepper
¼ - ½ tsp. dry mustard
2 tbsp. grated onion

Marinate vegetables for 1 or more hours. Refrigerate. Serve.

Poppyseed Dressing

(from Helen Corbitt and Neiman-Marcus)

Ingredients:

1 & ½ cup sugar
2 tsp salt
3 Tbsp onion juice
3 Tbsp poppyseeds
2 tsp dry mustard
2/3 cup vinegar
2 cup salad oil (preferable avocado or walnut)

Mix sugar, mustard, salt, and vinegar. Add onion juice and stir well. Add oil slowly, beating constantly. Beat until thick. Add poppyseed and mix well.

May use blender instead of mixer to combine. Store in a cool place or refrigerator, but do not freeze!

Fabulous dressing over fruit salads, but may also add avocado, celery, etc.

Marna L'Amie's Healthy Mayonnaise

In a small bowl, combine and beat these ingredients:

1 egg
Dash cayenne
½ teaspoon garlic
1 teaspoon Dijon mustard
½ teaspoon Worcestershire sauce
½ teaspoon salt
½ teaspoon pepper
2 teaspoon Xylitol (or raw sugar)
2 tablespoon fresh squeezed lemon juice

Pour into blender and add through hole in top... VERY SLOWLY... drop by drop to start with, while blending:

¼ cup Avocado oil
¼ cup Walnut oil
½ cup Olive oil...or...1/4 cup olive oil and 1/4 cup macadamia oil

(The slow addition makes an emulsion of the egg and oil.) After it thickens, put it in a jar in the refrigerator. It keeps a long time.

If you like, you may alter the amount of garlic, mustard, sugar, and Worcestershire to taste. Also, you may play with other healthy oils, such as sesame, pecan, or cashew.

Photos of Marna and Her Family

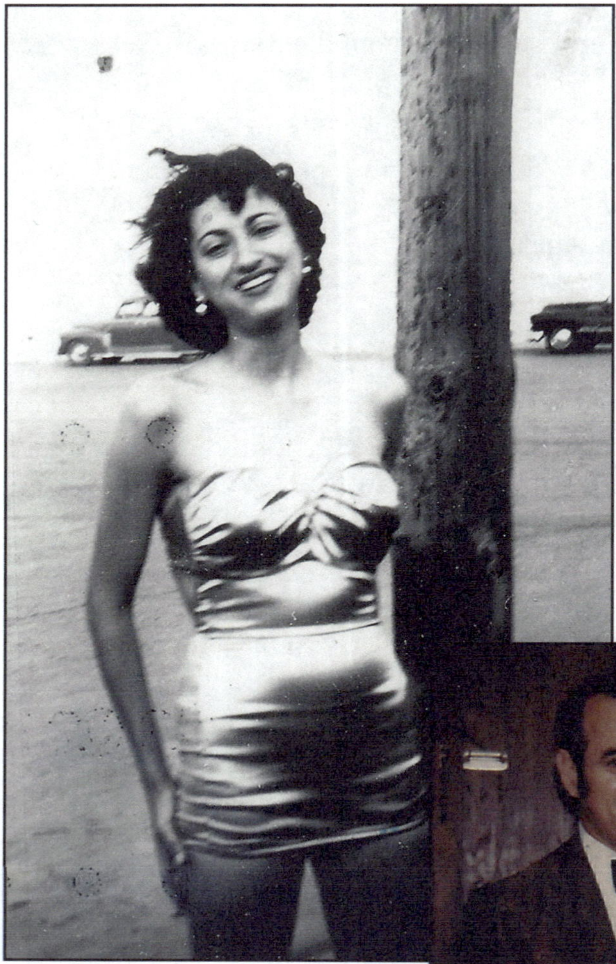

Young, dark-haired Marna in bathing suit. 1947, Galveston

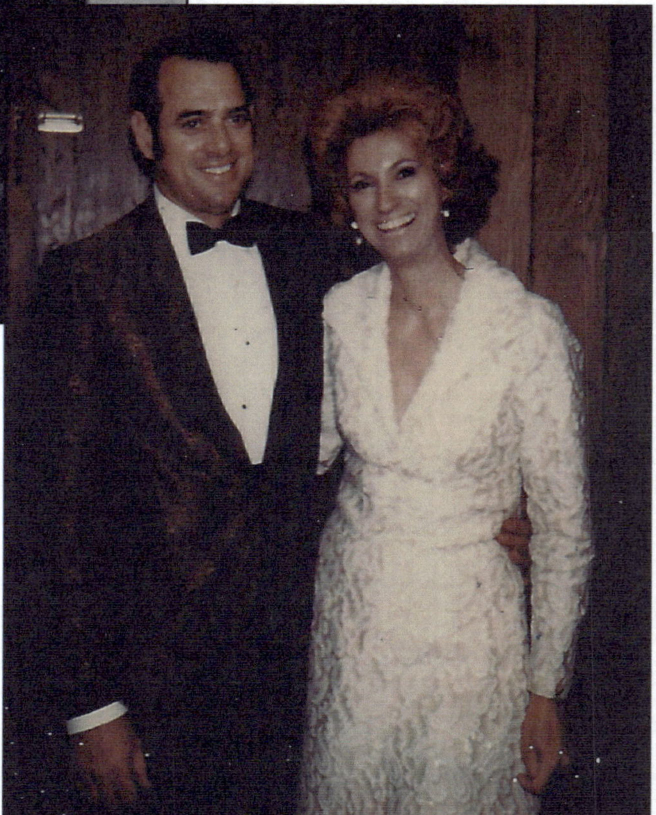

Mom and my father, Jack Franklin, dressed for ZBT fraternity party, 1972

Mom and one of her favorite cats 1980

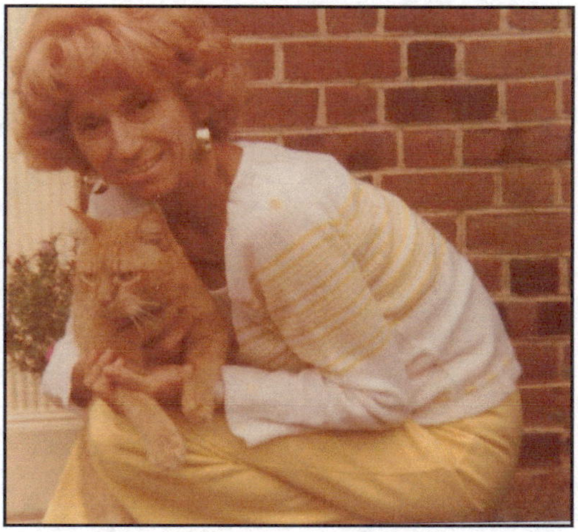

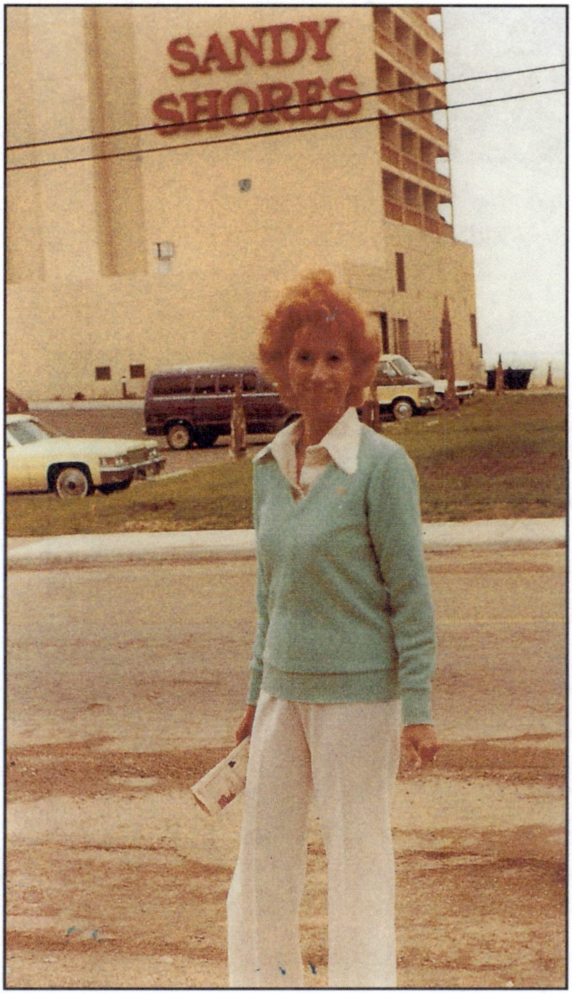

Mom at Sandy Shores, Corpus Christi, 1984

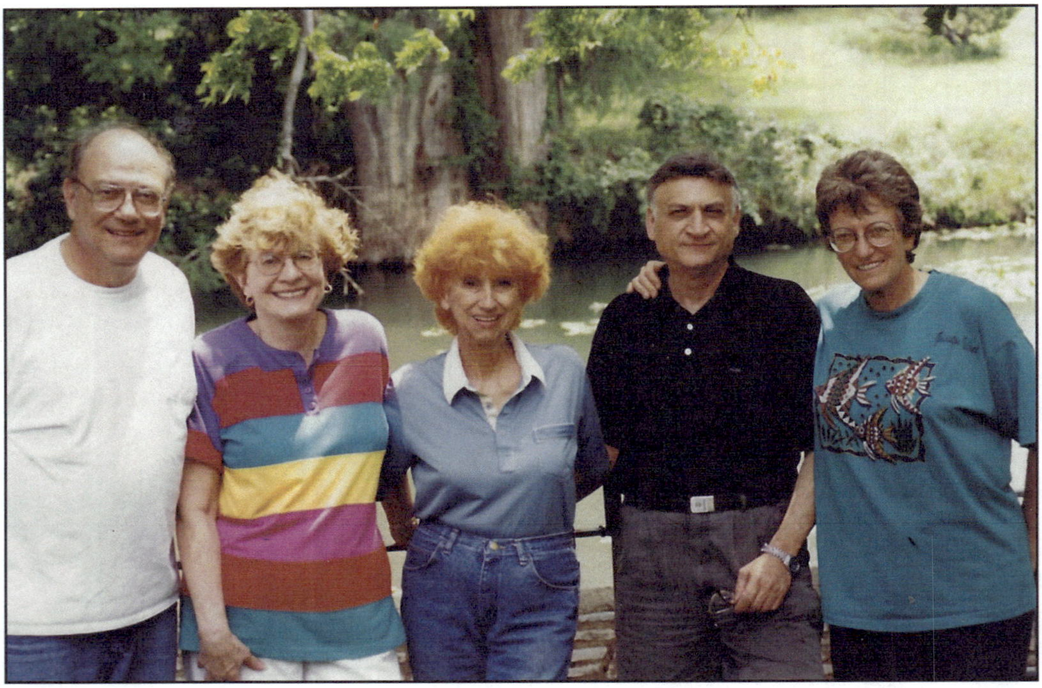

Mom with cousins, Joe Victor, Shirley Schaen, brother Jerry Robins, and cousin Rae Victor -- 70th birthday party, 1999

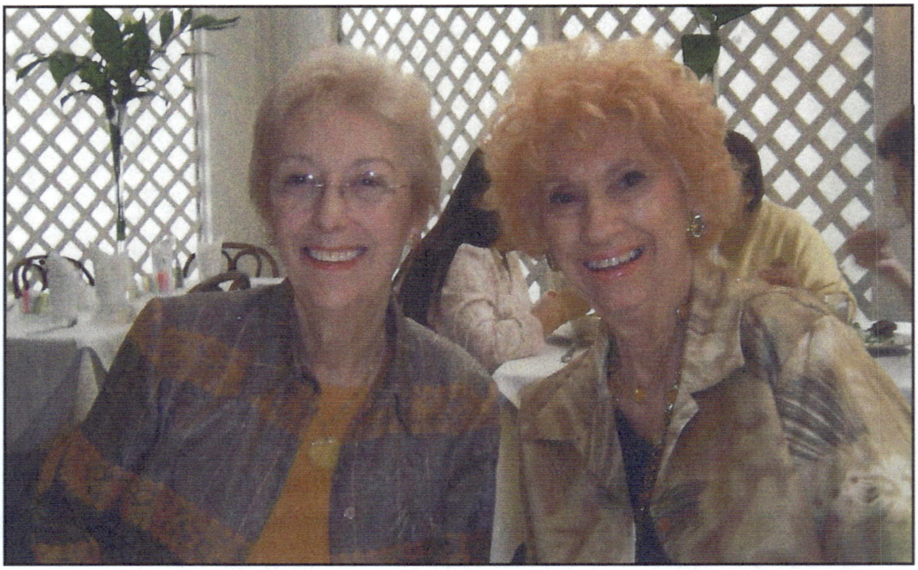

Mom with friend, Berniece in Brownsville, 2005

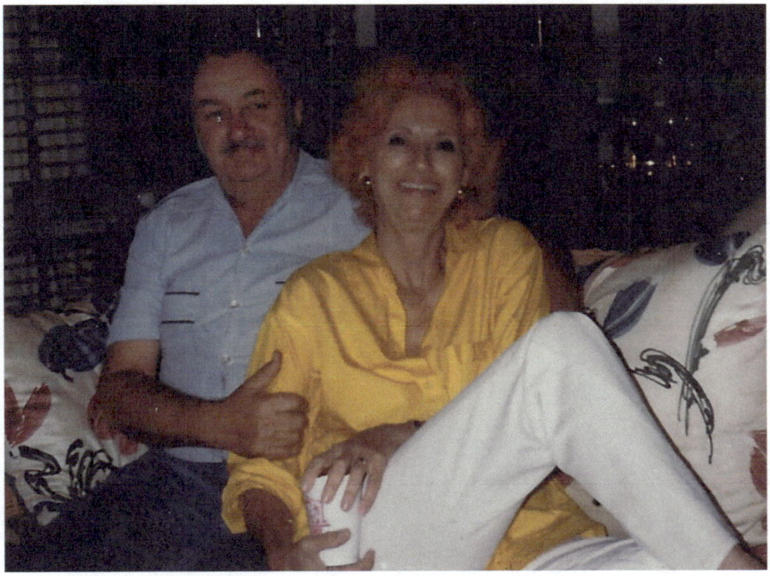

Mom relaxing with beloved husband, Bill L'Amie, 1986

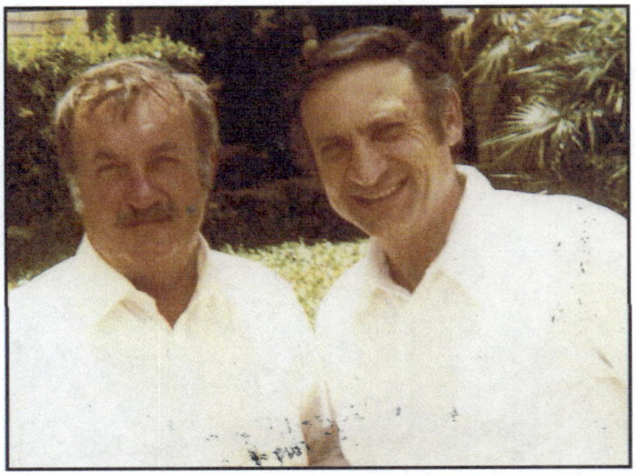

Bill L'Amie with Jerry Robbins 1980

Jerry Robbins 2019

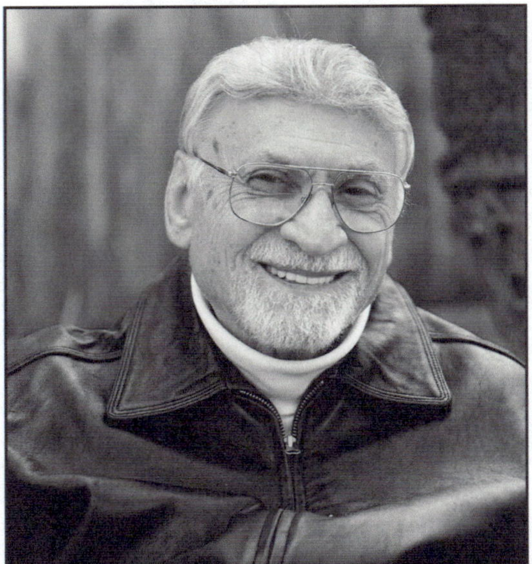

Acknowledgments

My mom, Marna L'Amie, died April 23, 2016. Since that time, much work has gone into compiling a collection of all her writings. Many friends and family members helped with this endeavor—collecting, organizing, and separating the plethora of articles and copies to make sure there was one of each, no matter the original location.

My friends Molly Hinds, Susan Smith, and my son-in-law Ryan Ties, all assisted. Susan Stark and Beth Brotherton gave me valuable advice on the "feel" of the book; Beth also helped with digitizing many of the original copies. Cathy Milner was invaluable at helping me with technical issues concerning copy and making suggestions for the final product. Cathy Ramsey, a talented artist, contributed the lovely sketches.

My husband Michael provided a supportive ear. And of course my three siblings, Lynda Furgatch, Reid Franklin, and Bram Franklin, for their suggestions and support.

Many thanks to the publisher, Cynthia Stone, and Treaty Oak Publishers. Cynthia was incredibly patient and helped make the daunting task of publication much easier.

Lastly, I would like to thank and acknowledge my uncle, Gerard Robins, who was the #1 fan of my mom's writings. He always encouraged her to publish her writings. It is my hope that this book will fulfill that wish.

Melanie Cox

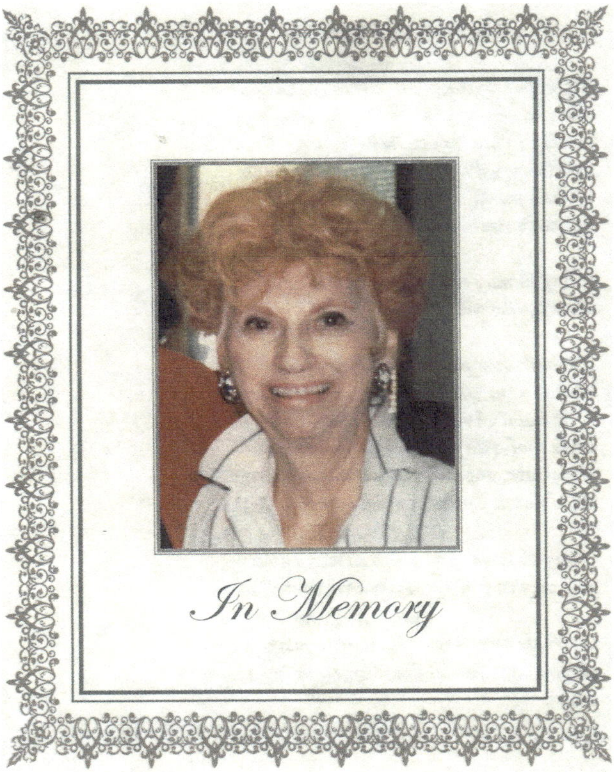

Made in United States
Cleveland, OH
05 November 2026

47763599R00114